Meta Fitness

YOUR THOUGHTS TAKING SHAPE

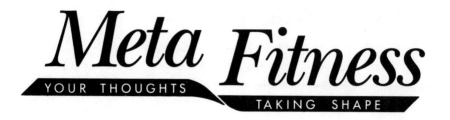

Meta Fitness
YOUR THOUGHTS   TAKING SHAPE

SUZY PRUDDEN

JOAN MEIJER-HIRSCHLAND

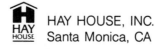

HAY HOUSE, INC.
Santa Monica, CA

Hay House, Inc.
501 Santa Monica Blvd.
Santa Monica, CA 90401

First Printing, June 1989

10 9 8 7 6 5 4 3 2 1

The author of this book does not dispense medical advice or prescribe the use of any technique as a form of treatment for physical or medical problems without the advice of a physician, either directly or indirectly. The intent of the author is only to offer information of a general nature to help you in your quest for physical fitness and good health. In the event you use any of the information in this book for yourself, the author and the publisher assume no responsibility for your actions.

Certain names in *MetaFitness, Your Thoughts Taking Shape* have been changed to protect the privacy of individuals who very kindly shared their stories in the hope of benefiting others.

ISBN 0-937611-48-4

Library of Congress Catalog Card No. 88-82803

Logo Design: Dan Eicholtz
Text Design: Gwen Rainey-Smith
Text Photos: Conrad Johnson
Suzy's Leotard: Flexatard® Gilda Marx®

Typesetting: Highpoint Type & Graphics, Claremont, CA
Printed and Bound in the United States of America by
Delta Lithograph Co. of Valencia, CA

DEDICATION

Although the dance is done,
It continues,
For it has only just begun.

People have asked me, "What helped you most during the time you went through your life changes? What kept you together when you lost your dream, when you thought there was no reason for life, no point to go on?"

The answer is simple: "My friends."

With their love and support I found that I could heal the wounds, create new dreams, and build a life filled with joy, excitement, and gratitude. I found that I could do anything. I dedicate this book to all those wonderful people with whom I laughed and cried and grew into the person I am today.

Special thanks to: Keith Buckler, Cherie Carter-Scott, Suzi Dean Finkelstein, Richard Foulk, Toni Galardi, Jonathan Goldhill, David Katzen, Margie Mirell, Rita Silverman, Emerald Dolphin Heart Star, and Lynn Stewart who loved, supported, and believed in me even when I had misplaced my belief in myself.

To: June Graham and Jim Spencer, David Gershon and Gail Straub, Ray Gottlieb and Marilyn Ferguson, Greg and Gail Hoag, Mariane Athey and Richard Karu, Herschell Freye and David Kaplan, Tim Karsten and Deborah Banker, Paula and Scooby Sorkin, Paul and Diana von Welanetz, and David La Chapelle, teachers and friends on my wonderous road to self-love and self-discovery.

To: Liz Brenner Dansiger, who introduced me to my California family and a new way of life.

To: Fred Anderson, Belva Bloomer, C.B. Brent, Mona Brookes, Jim Shannon, Rona Cherry, Imalda Collier, Jan Carolan, Donite Fried, Ruskin Germino, Jordan Glass, Susan Grossman, Katy Kasriel, Debra Judel Memorsky, Donna Sessler, Joe Sohm, Ruth Strassberg, Dyan Ullman, Shelly von Strunckel, Jamie Weinstein, Larry Weiss, George Yager, and Tyler Nelson, my dear friends spread over time.

To: Hana Cannon, Lin Laucella, Jim Leary, Dan Olmos, Linda Tomchin, Heather Williams, Laura Wilson, Steve Askew, Mary Jane Brandes, Kevin Pike, Gwen Rainey-Smith, and Jenny Collins, with whom I have worked at Hay House, Inc. I always felt loved and supported, understood and enjoyed by this team of beautiful people who took my manuscript and made a book.

To my sister, Petie (Joan Meijer-Hirschland), who wrote and created with me, who took over when I went blank, stepped aside when I was in full swing, who put up with me when I was impossible, and made me laugh when laughter did not exist.

To my son, Rob Sussman, who blessed my move to California and made it possible for me to be free.

And special thanks and much love to my dear friend and colleague, Louise L. Hay, who in her inimitable knowing, shrugged her shoulders and said, "Sure, why not? We could have fun with this." And MetaFitness began its journey into the world.

— Suzy Prudden

There have been many great teachers in my life during the past six years but none have had so profound and lasting an effect on me as my friends, Doug and Betts. Thank you.

— Joan Meijer-Hirschland

CONTENTS

INTRODUCTION

How I Created Meta Fitness

Until recently, my reputation in the fitness field was that of the fitness expert's expert. At the same time, my relationship with fitness had been one of struggle, starvation, self-abuse, and discomfort. Until 1981 I acted as if fitness, success, and self-abuse were synonymous. Although I taught that there is no gain in pain, I lived, until that time, a "no pain, no gain" existence. Finally my body and my mental stamina gave out. I just could not live my life in the same way anymore.

The change began in 1981 when I walked out on my husband and a way of life I thought I would live until I died. I came out of my eighteen-year marriage a battered woman. I felt battered, not simply by a brutal marriage and by my addictions to alcohol, Valium, and Soma, but by my continuing bulimia, slight bout with anorexia, and a conviction that I had to keep producing no matter what I was doing to my body and my mind. It took several years to make peace with my life and my body, and to reshape them the way I wanted them to be. What follows is the process I went through.

From 1981 to 1983, I struggled to keep myself in the fitness business, using methods that I had always known to be traditionally correct. But, after a lifetime of exercising, self-discipline, appalling hard work, and pain masked by drugs, I found myself unconsciously trying to destroy my career. My relationship with traditional fitness had been so painful that, subconsciously, I knew I had to leave the field.

Before I continue, it is important that I distinguish between MetaFitness, which I teach now, and traditional fitness, which I used to teach and which is taught throughout most of America. The difference is that MetaFitness works from the inside out: with the mind, feelings, and beliefs about the body and the self to create a positive relationship between them. The benefits of this approach are increased self-esteem, self-love, and self-appreciation. Traditional fitness, on the other hand, attempts to change the body and the self from the outside in. It does not take into account your underlying beliefs about your body or about the way you feel about yourself. In traditional fitness the underlying belief is that you must keep working to improve your exterior because you really are not okay. In MetaFitness the underlying belief is that you are always okay, you enjoy yourself, and you love and appreciate your body. You are never wrong in MetaFitness.

On a survival level, I used to think that teaching fitness was the only way that I knew how to make a living. On a deeper level, I did not want to teach anymore. On the one hand, I was ruining my business. On the other hand, I continued to try to work successfully in the field. The push-pull of leaving fitness while remaining a fitness expert was disorienting. Fitness was my identity but it no longer served me. In June 1981, I left a life of terror, physical and emotional abuse, loneliness, and self-depreciation. When I walked out on that life, a whole new world opened for me.

I felt like a genie let out of a bottle. I had very few outfits, other than leotards, to my name, so I went on a major five-year-long shopping spree. I began a process of learning to play, and allowed myself the joy in living that I had not experienced since I was a small child. I was tearing away at the fabric of my old being, but I had no way to put myself back together again. I had spent so many years masking my pain with drugs (Valium and Soma) that I had no foundation of self-esteem on which to build. Although I did not know it at the time, I was deeply depressed and dangerously self-destructive.

My mother, Bonnie Prudden, was extremely concerned for my well-being. She knew I needed tools to help me heal, and she suggested that I take a course in transformation which had helped her. Silva Mind Control started me on the path toward healing and self-love.

Confronting the monsters of my past was probably one of the most exciting and most painful things I have ever done. To my great surprise, I learned that I was not a horrible person. I also learned that I had a wonderful mind. (Until then I had always thought I was stupid.) Best of all, I learned that I had a great sense of humor. Suddenly I was surrounded by friends. It was a heady time.

I took course after course: Let Go and Live, The Empowerment Workshop Series, Opening the Heart, Money and You, The Mind Revolution, The Firewalk, Making Love Work, and The Loving Relationships Training. I spent weeks at The Omega and Esalen Institutes, and went on Vision Quests with David La Chapelle, camping out in the Colorado Rockies, the California deserts, and the rain forests and craters of Hawaii. I spent some time practicing Siddah Yoga, opened myself to Eastern philosophies, and even spent a week as a Samurai, playing George Leonard's Samurai War Game. Now I am working with Tim Piering in N.L.P. (Neuro-Linguistic Programming), Louise L. Hay, and Motivation Management Service, which created the Self-Esteem Workshop and Leadership and Consultants Trainings.

I learned that my belief system created my reality. I took personal responsibility for everything that had happened to me in the past, so that I could release it and never have to experience it again. Gradually I discovered the tools for learning who this person, Suzy Prudden, really is and I began to love myself.

I was still a fitness expert, yet I knew that I was not a traditional fitness expert. The problem was that I had no clear picture of what a fitness expert who was not traditional looked like. I knew that I had to teach people to heal their relationship with their bodies, but first I had to heal my own. The faint beginnings of a new kind of fitness took shape in my mind. In 1983, I gave in and sold the New York City exercise studio which had been my creation, my work place, and my identity for over eighteen years.

One day in 1986, I was invited to give a lecture in Los Angeles for an organization called The Inside Edge. I had been looking for a way to combine my understanding of metaphysics with my knowledge of physical fitness, knowing somewhere inside that this was my work. But I had no idea how to create it. As I began to speak, with no knowledge of what was to come, a whole new concept for being in one's body, MetaFitness, was born.

MetaFitness is the process of learning that self-love is a natural and healthy state of being. It is possible to look at your body and to find things you like about it, and to find ways that your body serves your life.

MetaFitness is a way of communicating with your body while you exercise, play sports, dance, or move in any way. You create a new relationship with your body if you listen to it, love it, honor it, and enjoy it. MetaFitness is magical. It's a way of passing through Alice's looking glass from the old programming, which taught us to focus on the negative, to a new programming which allows us to see the positive. I was brought up to believe that if I saw myself as beautiful and admitted liking myself, I was vain (which was bad). MetaFitness gave me permission to look in the mirror, see my beauty, and say, "Wow! You look great today!" and to believe it without guilt. Not only do I believe it, but I feel good about it.

1

HOW *MetaFitness* CAN WORK FOR YOU

"Your results are your teacher."
— *Sondra Ray*

MetaFitness utilizes affirmations, visualizations, and movement. It combines working with your body (the exterior) and working with your mind (the interior) to heal your relationship with yourself. Your body and the various components of your life (i.e., money, relationships, work, home, etc.) are the out-picturing of your inner self. As you heal your relationship with yourself, your relationship with your body and all other areas of your life begin to shift in a positive direction.

I believe that:

Your body is the physical manifestation of how you feel about yourself.

Everything "out there" (situations in your life) is a picture of what's going on "in here" (inside yourself and your belief system).

By healing your relationship with yourself, you heal your body and you heal your life.

Results such as long-term weight loss can occur, where weight loss has been difficult in the past. Changes in posture are possible, and permanent relief from pain can be experienced where no pathological causes are apparent (and even sometimes when there are pathological causes). Weight, pain, and posture problems are usually symptoms of blockages in your life. Look inside for the causes, heal them, and the symptoms are released. Your body serves as a weather vane for what's going on in the rest of your life. If you suddenly have shoulder pain, look at the burdens you carry in your life to see if they are heavier than usual. If you get a sore throat or laryngitis, look to see what you are not saying either to yourself or to an important person in your life. If you put on weight, look to see why you are protecting yourself and from what. Your body communicates what is going on before you can see it in your life. Until the cause is rooted out, the symptom will continue. So allow the symptom to lead you to the cause, then the cause can be healed.

In metaphysics, it is said, "What you focus on expands," and "Thought is creative. What you believe is true becomes true for you." If you focus on being fat by believing in it, by talking about it, by worrying about it, and by trying to do something about it, your body will respond by creating more fat.

For many people, fat is believed to be negative when actually it is something positive. Fat is a life-limiter, but it is also a great protector. It protects some people from unwanted sexual advances. For others, fat addresses the question, "What would happen if I really became as successful as I want to be? Could I handle it?" Fat can be a boundary-setter. Some people do not know how to protect themselves from the intrusions of others. They do not know how to say "no." In order to be protected, the body takes over and creates a boundary of fat to keep out anyone who gets too close too fast. The body says "no."

For me, extra weight cushioned me during times of extreme stress and feelings of fear as I left one way of life and created a new one. The body fat I developed limited my forward motion and gave me needed time out of the public eye to create and integrate my new work. I did not know it at the time, but the extra weight slowed me down and protected me from further burnout. Although I hated the extra weight, it was a blessing for me and for my career. I learned that fat is my body's way of protecting me during periods of drastic change; it keeps me safe when I am afraid. By reprogramming my mind during these fearful times, and by learning the reasons for my fears, I can let go of my excess weight and keep it off.

MetaFitness is not simply a process for weight loss. It can help you learn to like parts of yourself that, in some cases, you cannot even look at, to listen to your body and respect what it tells you, and to achieve good health and good feelings.

I found in my own life that I was programmed from childhood to ignore what my body told me: "Finish everything on your plate, other people are starving," so I ate when I wasn't hungry. "It's time for bed," but I wasn't sleepy. "Stop wiggling and sit up like a grown-up." "Stop acting like a child." In so many words and experiences, I was told that my body did not know anything, that it did not have any knowledge like the mind did, that it was merely a "thing." And what was worse, that I was this "thing," something to be tolerated and constantly improved.

As I grew up receiving these messages from the adult world, I stopped listening to my own messages. I forgot to pay attention, or even hear, when my body said it was satisfied, or tired. I forgot what it felt like to stop if I was in pain, or if I was becoming ill. My body became a thing to be dealt with rather than something with which to have a relationship.

Until recently, George, a friend and client of mine, was expected to spend the holidays every year with his in-laws with whom he did not get along. Two years ago, as he carried his family's luggage downstairs, he slipped, fell, and broke his leg. Needless to say, George did not spend those holidays with his in-laws. I thought it would have been a lot easier for him to say "no" in the first place, but he did not know that he could, so his body took care of the situation for him. He now spends the holidays traveling with his wife and children. They all have a wonderful time and his wife spends time with her parents when George is back at work. There is no more tension, and the holidays are a happy time of year, instead of something to be endured.

In 1986 my primary relationship was in trouble. Although I was very much in love with Jonathan, the man with whom I was living, I knew the relationship, as it was, was ending. Fearfully I kept quiet during difficult times, especially during the Christmas holidays. Because I was unwilling to express my feelings, I became ill with laryngitis and strep throat three days before Christmas. By New Year's Day I was feverish and bedridden (something that is rare for me). My intuition told me I had to speak; my fear kept me quiet. By the time all this occurred I had become aware that illness is the physical manifestation of something else going on in life. Since the throat represents communication, I asked myself the question, "What am I not saying?" The answer was clear: I had to tell Jonathan that our relationship was not working; I had to take the risk of hurting both of us. As soon as I stated my fears and my concerns to Jonathan, my body began to heal. Jonathan and I did separate, but we are still best friends, see each other often, and feel good about ourselves, each other, and our present relationship.

This incident taught me to pay attention to my body. Fatigue, pain, and injury occur when the self is denied, when you try to override personal will, and particularly when personal survival is at issue. When I listen to my body, pay attention to it, and follow its messages, I am healthy, have a great deal of energy, and can function comfortably in anything I undertake. The body is a "message machine."

I am still learning to recognize my body's signals that something is not working in my life. I still go off course sometimes, but it takes less time to get back on track each time.

Look at your own life. Can you see how your body lets you know when things are not working or when you are not following your instincts? The following exercises will help you learn to listen to yourself and honor your body with interest, ease, and gratitude.

EXERCISE: *Your Body As Your Teacher*

A. List two circumstances when you became ill or injured, and the emotional circumstances connected to these situations.

Example:
Christmas 1986, got sick twice during the holiday party season. Both times at a party (laryngitis and sore throat), both times twenty minutes after a fight with my boyfriend.

YOUR TURN

1. Back problem — Too much stress

2. Cold — too much going on.
Before trip — self sabotg

B. Can you see how in those situations you were not listening to your intuition, or doing what you knew was best for you?

Example:
Both times I wanted to speak up about the relationship, both times I kept quiet.

YOUR TURN

1. Not listening to message to slow down

2. Lot trusting in goodness

C. *Can you see how becoming ill or injured worked positively for you?*

Example:
Becoming sick showed me I was not being honest with myself. It allowed me to take better care of my life by dealing with the problem at hand and not letting it continue.

YOUR TURN

1. Yes, seeing a doctor

2. Awareness of amount of work.

D. *In looking back, what did you learn about yourself at the time? Where were you fearful or blocked in your life?*

Example:
I learned it was necessary to speak up for myself regardless of my fears.

YOUR TURN

1. Afraid of not being a good enough job.

2. Fearful of moving ahead

Your body and your mind have subtle ways of communicating with you. Learning to listen and respond to your body's messages will help you feel good all the time.

Your body plays an integral part in your life. It is not just the family car for trips around town. It is also the golden "all-terrain vehicle" in which you live and create adventures.

Your intuition is your guide. If honored, it will get you where you want to go, even if you are not consciously aware that you want to go there.

When you were a child you were fascinated with yourself. You loved every part of yourself unconditionally. You never got upset with yourself. You never made yourself wrong. You knew when you were hungry, angry, lonely, or tired, and you always asked for what you needed. Somewhere along the way you were taught that you did not know what your real needs were and that if you asked for what you wanted you were wrong. Growing up has become a process of giving up that wondrous, knowing child. MetaFitness will help you rediscover that child.

Affirmation

I am willing to hear
what my body is telling me.
I am open to learn from my body.

2

INTRODUCTION TO THE POWER
OF THOUGHT AND METAPHYSICS

"Ask, and it shall be given you;
Seek, and ye shall find,
Knock, and it shall be opened unto you."
— *Matthew 7:7*

*F*or many years, I believed there was someone or something doing things to me. My life did not work. I went on diets and gained back eleven pounds for every ten I lost. I applied for jobs I thought were perfect for me but did not get them. I ran out of money and could not make more. I could not seem to attract people into my life who supported and loved me as I wanted to be supported and loved. Then I began studying metaphysics, and my life took on a different perspective. This book starts with an introduction to metaphysics because without that vital piece of information, MetaFitness does not make sense. What I am presenting in this book is a theory that I have accepted as my belief system and as my way of life. By using this theory I have been able to change every single aspect of my life in a positive direction, especially my relationship with my body.

Metaphysics means: beyond the physical or material.

The basic premise of metaphysics, as we understand it today is: Thought is creative. What you believe to be true, both on a conscious level where you see it, and on a subconscious level where you cannot, becomes your reality.

In other words, you create your life with your thoughts, your beliefs, and the way you express yourself with the words you choose. Your life is 100 percent your responsibility, no matter what other people may be doing to you. The bad news is, there is no one out there to blame. The good news is, because your life is 100 percent your responsibility, you are in charge (not a victim) and you can choose to change it. That may not make sense at first, but as you begin to practice this principle, as you see it work, it gets easier. It is a very powerful concept. What makes it powerful is that it works.

How Your Mind (Meta) Works:
The Monitor, or Critic, or Judge

There is a part of the brain, or the mind, which monitors. It is quite separate and distinct from the practical part, that part of the brain which supervises the body's functions and gets us to appointments on time. The monitor talks incessantly: "You're right." "You're wrong." "You're good." "You're bad." "You're pretty." "You're ugly." "He's nice." "He's good for you." "Yes." "No." "Do." "Don't." "But. . ." "Now." "Later." "Never." "Why?" "Why did he say that to me?" "Just look at her hair!" "Blondes have more fun." "Men never make passes at girls who wear glasses." "Oh my God, look at your thighs!" It talks and chatters all through the day.

I call it my critical voice, because whether I am judging myself or judging someone else, **my mind is judging me**. According to this belief system, all the mind ever hears is "I"; **I=I, You=I, They=I, He=I, She=I**. The mind cannot judge in others what it cannot perceive in itself.

I have learned to pay attention when I judge other people, because what I am judging in them may be something I need to look at about myself. This can be tricky at first, but once you catch on to the idea, it is very freeing. Of course, the good part is, when you praise other people your mind also hears it as "I," so you are also praising yourself. If I really want to make myself feel great I write a letter to someone I love, telling them all the things I find wonderful about them. It makes both of us feel good.

Most people believe that their mind chatter, those thoughts that are in their head much of the day, their critical voice, is real. They give it control over their lives. I certainly did. They think that because they have a thought, then it must be right. I used to believe that my critical voice was like the voice of God; it knew something I did not know. But recently, I realized that I made up the critical voice. It came from my brain, my mind, my way of thinking. It is not real, but it used to sit like the devil on my shoulder and tell me all the things I was doing wrong. Now I try to prevent my critical voice from hurting me by being quicker than it is and more aware of it than I used to be. Although I cannot shut it up completely, more and more often I can make it quieter. What a relief.

You may ask, "How do I get my critical voice to become quiet?" By becoming aware. Listen to what your critical voice is saying to you.

Pretend you burned the toast at breakfast. Your critical voice starts to yell at you. It will set up a barrage of chatter about how bad or wrong you are. You have a choice here. You can believe it, and therefore believe you are bad and wrong, or you can simply notice that you burned the toast. You will probably make new toast no matter how you feel about yourself. It makes more sense to feel okay rather than bad and wrong.

It may take practice, so keep noticing. There will come a time when you have a clear understanding that the critical voice is merely mind chatter and you do not have to let it rule you. Whenever you hear it talking to you, thank it for sharing and release your reaction to it. Just remember, the first step is knowing you are okay.

Part of the process of changing your body involves identifying your mind chatter about it. This can help you find out how you really feel about your body on a subconscious level.

The Subconscious Creator

There is another hidden piece of the mind-puzzle. In addition to the practical part of the brain and the monitor, there is a part of the brain of which many people are not consciously aware: the subconscious. The subconscious mind is like a black hole. Black holes are collapsed stars. They have the most powerful gravitational pull in the universe, yet we cannot see them. Black holes were first identified mathematically, then verified by the influence they exerted on surrounding planets and systems.

Like the black hole, the subconscious cannot be seen. We only know it is there because we see it in action. I sometimes use carbon monoxide as a metaphor for the subconscious. Carbon monoxide is a colorless, odorless, and tasteless gas, but it can kill. The subconscious is colorless, odorless, and tasteless, yet it has near total control over the direction of our lives. The subconscious mind colors our conscious desires.

The subconscious is the real power that controls everything in our lives. It is the power behind the throne. It is our hidden computer program. We have stored information and made decisions about the way everything works based on things we have heard and seen starting at birth and even before. This programming, these beliefs, color our lives.

Identifying Subconscious Thoughts and Decisions

Our subconscious mind is so subtle that the only way to identify what it is thinking is by looking at the results, the way our thoughts play out in our lives.

Everything on the outside (situations and experiences) is merely a picture of what is going on inside. To identify the patterns of our lives, it is necessary to look at the results.

Helen, a client of mine, has been on ten thousand diets. (That is possibly a slight exaggeration, but she says it feels like ten thousand.) Every time she goes on a diet, she loses weight. As soon as she goes off her diet, she gains back the weight she lost, plus a few pounds.

There are many scientific theories about weight loss and weight gain. One theory talks about our primitive past which created a feast and famine survival mechanism in our bodies in the days when there was no refrigeration or reliable food sources. Another theory says the more you diet the more your body adjusts, needing less and less food and burning calories slower and slower. Eventually, eating what used to be normal becomes too much. Still another theory says if you created an abundance of fat cells as a child, these fat cells will lie in wait to be filled as an adult. They sit there, waiting to become full, and you can never get rid of them except through liposuction.

All these theories make sense, and they all work as far as the results are concerned: they explain why it is difficult to lose weight. But what if your subconscious is really behind the scene? What if your subconscious has a reason for you to be fat? For example, what if your subconscious has decided that fat is safe and thin is not?

Helen walks around New York City feeling absolutely safe in her overweight body. Men used to make catcalls and accost her in the subway when she was slender. Now that she is heavy, she feels almost invisible. Helen feels safe when she is fat. Using MetaFitness, Helen learned how to feel safe when she is slender. By following the examples in this book, Helen discovered the reasons why she felt safer fat. She committed to make a change, set her goals, and then followed through with a MetaFitness program she designed for herself. Subconsciously, Helen no longer has to be fat to feel safe.

The Powerful Inner Voice

There is a part of us which "knows" what is right and "knows" what we need to do. It is not a thinking part, not a chattering part, not a dictating part. It is a knowing part. Call it intuition, a deep inner-knowing, a gut reaction. Call it the still small voice. It always knows what is our right choice. It is our guide. Many people believe it is God's way of communicating with us. All too often we discount this voice until **after** a disaster has occurred.

During the past few years, listening to this inner voice has enabled me to create a very exciting and fruitful life. People sometimes will ask me why I do things and I can only answer, "It feels right." When I am willing to listen to my inner voice and not be afraid, I always know what to do, even without a reason or when it looks risky and makes no logical sense.

A few years ago, Mary, one of my clients, went to work as a temporary secretary for a small public relations firm. Although she had no real interest in public relations, the owner of the business said he recognized her intelligence and wanted to train her to become a public relations account executive, earning lots of money. One month into her employment she recognized that this man was emotionally abusive, and he was not training her as he promised. Although she stayed on the job, Mary's survival instinct was triggered. Her inner voice told her to leave, but her critical voice or mind chatter told her that he was her boss and so he must be right. Her critical voice became a partner in the abuse while her inner voice cried, unheeded, for her to leave. It was not until Mary became physically ill that she finally left the job. Her body responded to her inner voice even though she, herself, could not.

In retrospect, Mary can remember that when she first started the job her inner voice said, "This is going to be very bad and you ought to leave." But her critical voice, or mind chatter, said, "You always run away from difficult situations, you can make this one work. Think of the money. At least you will have a career." Her body made the difference; getting sick was her body's way of making Mary listen to her inner voice.

Most of us have experienced our inner voice, or intuition, at work. Chances are it has been guiding you for years. How often have you said, "Something told me that was not a good idea," or "I knew I ought to have done it. I know every time, but I do not always listen."

The difference between the critical voice and the inner voice is that the critical voice usually speaks about fears or survival, powerlessness, or negativity. It also sounds very logical. The inner voice often has no logic at all. It is just a quiet knowing, it has no judgment, it just is. It is not attached to fear but very often appears to be the thing you least want to hear because it appears to be the hardest choice, although, in the long run, the best choice.

In the beginning it may be necessary to practice listening for your inner voice. Just begin by noticing it and seeing what happens when you follow it and when you do not. You may have to identify your "knowing" after the fact.

It might seem like you know not to do something, but you do it anyway, with an unpleasant result which could have been avoided if you had listened to your inner voice. Or you may have an idea and although it seems ridiculous at the time, because you have no real reason to follow through on it, you do it anyway and the results are phenomenal. Listen to your inner voice.

EXERCISE: *Recognizing Your Inner Voice*

A. Write down an example of when you intuitively knew something. (Hearing a voice may be misleading. Usually it is a feeling or a knowing.)

Example:
On a recent trip to New York, I had to buy some rain boots. For some reason I knew that I would find the perfect boots at Alexander's. I never shop at Alexander's and yet I knew I would find the boots there.

YOUR TURN

_____

_____

_____

_____

B. Did you listen to your inner knowing at the time?

Example:
No. Although I "knew" I would find the boots at Alexander's, and it was only two blocks away, I went forty blocks to Macy's.

YOUR TURN

_____

_____

_____

_____

C. What happened when you did not listen to your inner voice?

Example:
I did not find the boots at Macy's, or anywhere else, and I walked forty blocks in the rain.

YOUR TURN

_____

_____

_____

_____

D.   Can you see how you could have done it differently?

Example:
Yes. I could have gone to Alexander's in the first place, which my inner knowing told me to do.

YOUR TURN

_____

_____

_____

_____

E.   What would have happened if you had listened and acted?

Example:
If I had listened I would have gone to Alexander's in the first place. I finally did go to Alexander's where I found the rain boots. I could have had dry feet and boots in twenty minutes instead of wet feet, tired legs, a grumpy disposition, and ruined leather boots.

YOUR TURN

_____

_____

_____

_____

F.   Can you see a positive result from listening to your inner voice?

Example:
Had I listened, I would have saved time and had what I wanted immediately.

YOUR TURN

_____

_____

_____

_____

This book will show you the difference between "mind chatter" and the "still small voice," the "critical voice" and "the inner knowing." You will learn how to listen to that still small voice, even when it seems silly. The written techniques will help you begin to identify your subconscious beliefs by looking at the results those beliefs cause in your life. This awareness will help you reprogram your life on a subconscious, as well as conscious, level and enable you to achieve the goals that have eluded you.

Mind chatter is very subtle. It is a tool of the subconscious mind. It colors your thoughts with hidden messages. The subconscious mind, with the chatter that it uses to communicate, is like the highly sophisticated computer in the movie *War Games*. The computer begins playing a game called War, which it is programmed to win. America is brought to the brink of World War III because no one in authority knows that the computer is playing a game, no one knows that the computer is in charge. Sometimes our lives are similar to that movie: We may not realize that our every thought is colored by something with a hidden agenda—our subconscious.

When you learn to recognize some of your subconscious patterns, and play the "game of life" consciously, you can reprogram your subconscious and, in so doing, your body, so your relationship with your body will change.

Your relationship with your body parallels your relationship with your partner, significant other, money, with work, family, everything in your life. It is the physical manifestation of your relationship with yourself and your beliefs.

Think of your subconscious beliefs as pillars holding up the whole structure of your life. There are actually very few bottom lines, or support pillars, in anyone's life. The thoughts that affect one thing will affect all other things. If you can figure out what your subconscious mind is telling you, you will suddenly see what is keeping you from having a body or life that you can love, or loving the body or life you have.

Examples of bottom-line beliefs are: "I am not good enough." "I am unwanted." "I am unlovable." "I never have enough." "I always hurt people." "People always hurt me." "I am a victim." "I am bad." But, underlying most bottom-line beliefs is one belief: "I am not good enough."

I will show you how to overcome the "not good enough" belief as it refers to your body. As you develop a belief in your body that you can accept, you will develop a relationship with yourself that feels good. This relationship will spill over into all your other relationships. The final result will be the creation of a successful, happy life, which you want and which you so richly deserve.

EXERCISE: *Why Things Go Right or Wrong in Your Life*

The way to identify the subconscious part of the mind is to become aware of the things that consistently go right or wrong in your life.

A.   Write three things that consistently go right in your life (e.g., you never have to wait for a bus or subway train, you always find a parking space, you always wear a size eight no matter how much you eat).

Example:
1. I always find the perfect home to live in. It is always beautiful and exactly what I want and need.
2. I always have enough money to pay my bills and support myself comfortably.
3. My friends are extremely intelligent and very successful. They are always the leaders in whichever group I happen to join.

YOUR TURN

1. _____

_____

_____

2. _____

_____

_____

3. _____

_____

_____

B.   Write three things that consistently go wrong in your life (e.g., you always have to wait for a bus or subway, you never find a good parking space, you are always a size sixteen or eighteen no matter how little you eat).

Example:
1. Other people know more than I do and therefore I am not as successful as I'd like to be.
2. I never seem to be able to get my weight below 125 pounds.
3. I never can have a relationship and a successful career at the same time.

YOUR TURN

1. _____

_____

_____

2. _____

_____

_____

3. _____

_____

_____

C.   Write down your beliefs. Be willing to acknowledge that you have a belief (that you always or never wait, or find a parking space, or gain weight). Can you see that you make that belief stronger by constantly thinking it or saying it aloud to other people? For example: "I can't ever seem to lose weight," or "I'll never be a size eight," or "I barely eat a thing and I still gain weight," or "I wish I could, but it'll never happen." Are you willing to see that the belief is there, and that it appears to be based on observation of established fact?

What always works for you?

Example:
1. I believe that I can always have the home of my dreams.
2. Although I fear that I will not have enough money, I know that I always will.
3. Because of my intelligence and leadership ability, I always attract intelligent people, who I feel are leaders, to be my friends.

YOUR TURN

1. _____

_____

_____

2. _____

_____

_____

3. _____

_____

_____

D.   *What does not work out for you?*

Example:
1. I believe I do not know enough to be a true success.
2. I cannot weigh less than 125 pounds and remain safe and grounded.
3. If I have a relationship, I have to give up my career.

YOUR TURN

1. _____

_____

_____

2.

_____

_____

_____

3.

_____

_____

_____

It Is Thought, Not Fact, That Comes First

- First you think that you never have to wait for a bus;
- Then you never have to wait for a bus;
- Then you notice that you never have to wait for a bus;
- Then it becomes a fact that you never have to wait;
- Then you begin saying that you never have to wait for a bus, which reinforces the thought that you never have to wait for a bus.

- First I think I can have the house of my dreams;
- Then I begin to always find the house I dream of;
- Then I notice that I always find the perfect house;
- Then it becomes a fact that I always find the perfect house;
- Then I begin saying that I always find the perfect house, which reinforces the thought that I always find the perfect house.

The concept that the thought comes first is one of the most powerful concepts in the world today, because if the thought comes first, then you can change your reality by changing your thoughts. **You can be in charge of your life.** Replace that first thought with a new idea and you can create a different reality. You can literally change your life. If you have the thought that you are fat, you can change that thought. When you do, your body and actions will follow the new instructions. It takes practice and work. It does not happen just by saying it once to yourself and expecting results. It does take time, but it works.

While working on your relationship with your body, you will develop a new relationship with success, with money, and with people. The subconscious underpinning is the same for the body as it is for all things.

Affirmation

I am 100 percent in charge
of my life and my body.
They can be whatever I want them to be.

3

THE METAPHYSICS OF BODY PARTS

*"The Spirit inspires, the Will responds
to inspiration, and together they experience
in the Body. Body is the manifestation
of Spirit and Will."*
— *channeled by Ceanne DeRohan*

Sometimes the only way to figure out what thoughts are governing your life is to look at the results of those thoughts (your life as you are living it) and work backward. If you tell yourself that you are a successful businessperson and your business keeps going Chapter 11, maybe you have a subconscious belief that you will fail.

The body is a reflection of what is going on in your life, particularly for things you do not see clearly. For example, pain in the neck represents stubbornness or inflexibility, the stomach is a barometer of how you digest and assimilate new ideas. The body may know weeks, months, or even years before your mind allows you to recognize that your life is not in perfect harmony.

In this chapter you will learn to identify body problems (not primarily problems of disease) and what they may mean in terms of life decisions and subconscious beliefs. For some of you, many of these suggestions may hit the nail on the head; for others, only one or two may make sense. It is only a starting point, but it will help you determine what works for you.

What It Means When Something Does Not Work

Whenever I experience pain or illness (body sensations), I try to find what may be causing or contributing to the problem by looking at my life. Usually, I am out of step. When I adjust the way I am living, including allowing a little healing time, I become well.

A couple of years ago, I was very stuck in the direction my life was taking—or was not taking—and I was unable to move forward in my career, or even recognize what I wanted to do with my life. I had dreams of creating a whole new form of fitness but was afraid of how the public would receive my new information. I recognized that I liked being out on the leading edge, yet I was afraid to risk being out there. I did not know how to bridge the gap between traditional physical fitness practices and the metaphysical beliefs I understood. While I could not see where I was going, I was absolutely clear that traditional fitness was no longer working for me. Every day was a battle between the safety of what I had always done and the knowledge that I could no longer do it.

Unable to work, I went horseback riding with a friend. She needed help with a new and very difficult horse. An excellent rider, I volunteered to get the horse to move past the places where he continued to balk. (As I write this I am just now aware of the parallel between moving the horse forward in his training and moving myself forward in my work.) An epic battle ensued between the horse and me. He refused to move past the imaginary line he did not want to cross. I insisted he go forward. Finally, he reared up, fell over backward and landed on my leg, pinning me underneath his body; I was trapped between a six-foot-high brick wall and the horse. Fortunately, he got up moving away from the wall rather than toward it, where I was lying. Although in extreme pain, I followed my training, got back on the horse, and moved him past where he was stuck.

That evening, I saw my acupuncturist, who thought my leg might be broken and suggested I get it x-rayed. I agreed. It was becoming increasingly difficult to tolerate the sharp pains I felt each time I moved.

I was very frightened, and yet, somehow I realized that the injury was a clue, telling me to look at my life. I knew that when I figured out what it represented and took appropriate action, I would heal.

I opened Louise L. Hay's book, *You Can Heal Your Life*, and read about the lower leg. It said, "Fear of the future. Not wanting to move." There it was in black and white, exactly what was going on in my life, and it was my black and blue leg that was telling me about it. Before, if I had injured my leg, I would simply have gone to the doctor, gotten a cast, and waited for it to heal. This time I used a different approach. I had nothing to lose by believing that my injured leg represented my inability to move forward in life. At that moment, I made up my mind to commit to my future, to move forward in my career, to get off the fence, and to chance being on the leading edge of a new concept. I felt a rush of energy, a palpable shift of some kind. I placed my leg on a pillow so that it would be comfortable while I slept, turned off the light, and prayed it was not broken.

When I see a movie, I am aware that everything on the screen is there for a purpose. Every detail advances the plot and is a clue to the audience about what is going on. But the characters often miss the clues, even when they see them, because their attention is focused elsewhere.

We are all stars of our own movies. We have as much difficulty seeing what is obvious to others, or obvious by hindsight as any character of a movie. Nothing in our lives is there without a reason. Everything has meaning when we are willing to look at it and when we have the tools to understand.

In the morning, I woke up, afraid that my leg was broken. I removed the covers and tentatively stepped out of bed. I felt no pain, and there was no swelling, just a faint discoloration where the injury had been the day before (to remind me that it was not an illusion). I knew at that moment that I had healed my leg by committing to moving forward in my life. I knew there was no going back.

The use of metaphysical tools enabled me, with my own mind, to heal my body and begin to heal my life. This experience showed me how responsive my body is to the power of my mind. It also showed me how powerful my willingness to commit to myself can be.

I realized how fast I could move in my life when I understood the messages my body gave me, and then took action. The form of the message was not as important as the fact of the message. The fact of the message was less important than my willingness to act. Action was less important than the energy of my commitment. My commitment to my life healed my body. That is the message of MetaFitness.

Each of the twelve major body parts functions as a mirror or metaphor for what is going on in your life. We will look at what these areas represent, as well as your skin and muscles, in general, and finally, four basic physical problems.

FACE

Your face represents what you show the world. It also represents what you hide from yourself and the world. Inner feelings, even the ones not conscious to you, very often appear on the face. When you have difficulties with parts of your face, you may want to look at what you are hiding or withholding.

Eyes

Your eyes represent what you see in the world, what you see in your life, and your attitudes toward that which you see. They represent your willingness to look at all of life, as well as your ability to look honestly at yourself, your relationships, home, work, money, etc. When you have difficulties with vision, try looking at what you do not want to see.

Nose

Your nose represents self-recognition and how you see yourself in the world—whether or not you want to be noticed or whether you want to be invisible. Your nose also represents how comfortable you are with yourself as part of the world and your ability to know what you want and to get what you need. A runny nose, for example, may be expressing a "crying" need for help.

Cheeks

Your cheeks represent your feelings of shame and not being good enough. Notice how you "feel" when you embarrass yourself and what your cheeks do in reaction to that feeling. Blemishes or scars tell you of your inner feelings of inadequacy, guilt, or shame. Perhaps feelings of guilt, shame, or not being good enough came first and the blemishes or scars are merely the outward expression of them.

Mouth

Your mouth represents taking in new ideas and nourishment. It is the gateway for expression as well as reception. Pain in the mouth often represents confusion or an inability to make a decision, or to process what you are learning, experiencing, or trying to express.

Chin

Your chin represents power or powerlessness in the world. How you hold your chin as well as its shape and size can tell you about your inner feelings regarding power and your relationship to it. Overly sensitive people, for instance, may continually tuck their chin under as if to protect it from what they fear may hit it. Blemishes on the chin may represent an unwillingness to assume full power, or a need to overcome obstacles to achieve full power.

Ears

Your ears represent your capacity and willingness to hear, to take in and assimilate information. They also tell you if you are comfortable with your surroundings, or what the people or situations in your life are "telling" you. Earaches often represent anger and frustration. Poor hearing may represent an unwillingness to take in new information. Or it may mean you are turned off to those close to you and do not want to hear them.

Hair

Your hair represents your ability to trust life and allow and acknowledge your feelings. Hair also represents being comfortable with your sexuality—

your femininity or masculinity—and your sensuality, and whether or not you are comfortable allowing yourself to feel and fully enjoy your physical body.

Baldness

Baldness represents fear and tension in life. It represents trying to control rather than trusting in life's process. It is almost as if you try so hard to hold on and control your life with your mind that you have cut off the circulation to the roots of your hair. (This, of course, is an image, not a statement of fact.)

Some people choose to be bald by shaving their heads. This may be a statement of "I am in control," when underneath there is the fear and feeling of being out of control. Or it may mean they surrender to not having control and enjoy the freedom of letting go.

NECK AND SHOULDERS

Neck

Your neck represents balance and flexibility. It serves as the conduit for information between the mind and the body. It represents the ability to perceive what surrounds you, what you just left, what you are going through, and where you are going. The neck represents looking at all sides of a situation. When you have a stiff neck, you may not be looking honestly at your life and/or you may be unwilling to be flexible in dealing with your life situations.

Shoulders

Your shoulders represent that which carries and supports. When there is pain in the shoulders you may be feeling burdened by your life. Your shoulders also represent your willingness to know or not to know. Notice your attitude toward yourself when you shrug your shoulders. Is it all right for you not to know? And when you do know something, are you attached to that knowledge? Shoulders also represent the way you deal with authority. A higher right shoulder means you deal overtly, a higher left shoulder means you deal covertly.

ARMS

Upper Arms

Your upper arms represent the capacity to embrace all that life has to offer. They represent the joy or discouragement you feel with the experiences of your life. Pain in your upper arms may mean you are holding yourself back from experiencing life fully. If you are afraid to live life fully, to really go for it, you may experience weight gain in your upper arms.

Elbows

Your elbows represent changing directions in life and accepting new experiences. If you feel stiffness or pain in your elbows you may be uncomfortable with change. Holding on too tightly to the old may manifest in elbow discomfort. Tennis elbow is a sure sign of rigidity.

Lower Arms

Your lower arms represent your ability to balance and hold that which you carry in life. They also represent your ability to take the time necessary to center yourself while juggling many things at once. You may experience pain or weakness in your lower arms when you feel you do not have the capacity to handle everything.

Wrists

Your wrists represent your ability to move with ease while handling your life. They also represent how you move in your life: fluidly, rigidly, lightly, with ease, or with difficulty. Your wrists also represent how you accept or reject pleasure in your life.

HANDS AND FINGERS

Hands

Your hands represent the ability to grasp and handle life. They also represent the limitations we put on ourselves, our skillfulness and dexterity at managing things. Pain in the hands means trying to "handle" everything for yourself and others beyond your capacity, without allowing the emotions that you feel to be expressed. Notice how people express things with their hands. When emotions are not expressed or are turned inward, the hands may experience pain or discomfort. (Among other things, arthritis is a manifestation of resentment. When feelings are not expressed, resentment builds in the body. As the hands are tools of expression, arthritis often occurs in the hands of people who feel thwarted or resentful in their lives.) How you hold your hands indicates what you are willing to express and how you want others to see you. Fists indicate anger and resentment, a wishy-washy handshake expresses a blase attitude toward life, pain can mean feelings of unexpressed resentment.

Fingers

Your fingers represent the details in life.

The Thumb represents your personal will and whether or not you want to be where you are, either in a certain situation or in life in general. It also represents intellect and worry.

The Index Finger represents your ambition, your ego and fear, willingness to follow your intuition, skill at handling money and projects (business), and leadership ability.

The Middle Finger represents your sense of right and wrong, your integrity with yourself and others, your search for inner truth, introspection, your standards for behavior in the world, your anger and sexuality.

The Ring Finger represents your creative power, grief, and self-expression. It also represents your ability to merge with others or to remain autonomous.

The Little Finger represents communication, pretending, and family relationships.

THE BACK

Upper Back

Your upper back guards the heart. It represents safety and support. It also represents love and trust. When there is pain in the upper back, often it means fear, either of giving or receiving love or not being able to trust either oneself or someone else, and most importantly, not trusting the Universe (your Higher Power). Pain in the upper back means fear of betrayal. "Stabbed in the back" is an American idiom representative of that fear, as is, "Don't turn your back on him."

A key concept in back problems is willingness to receive. If you have upper back problems, look at your willingness to receive love and support. Look at your willingness to trust. Look at your belief about whether or not love is or can be there for you. Clearing up upper back problems is a major leap in faith.

Mid-Back

Your mid-back represents feelings of guilt and being stuck in the "gunk" of life. It also represents fear of being hemmed in or taken advantage of. You might want to look at what guilt you are carrying around that you no longer need, or if you feel stuck in your life, or if there are persons or responsibilities you are "carrying" that you no longer need or want to carry.

Lower Back

Your lower back represents support. In this culture, support is represented by money and real property. Pain in the lower back occurs when there is a deep subconscious fear that there is not enough. In most cases the fear revolves around money. This is a tricky one. A person may appear to have plenty of money, and may even be a millionaire, but the deep-seated fear and the pain is still there. Fear is an illusion.

Lower back problems may mean a lack of trust that there will always be enough in life. Fear and trust cannot exist in the same space.

CHEST AND BREASTS

The Chest

Your chest represents your ability to take in both love and life. It represents your ability to feel safe in love. The chest houses both the lungs and the heart, two major life centers. Without the ability to take in oxygen or to pump blood through your body, your body dies. Pain in the chest, depending on where it is located, can be associated with fear, guilt, anger, repression, rigidity, and grief.

The chest is also the center of giving. It is the site where children are nurtured by their mothers. When people comfort or love each other they embrace one another to their chests. When the ability to give or receive is blocked, pain in the chest (heart or lungs) may follow.

The Breasts

Your breasts represent nurturing of self and others. They also represent nourishment both physically, as in food, and emotionally, as in feelings. When one does not get enough nourishment either from others or from oneself, one may experience breast discomfort. When a woman does not enjoy her role as a nurturer, or finds herself nurturing others at her own expense, she may experience breast problems, even cancer. Breasts also represent a woman's feelings about her own femininity and sensuality.

MIDRIFF AND WAIST

Midriff

Your midriff represents how you deal with your emotions, with ease or difficulty, with confidence or fear. It holds your major secondary vital organs: your liver, spleen, kidneys, pancreas, top of the large bowel, top of the small bowel, stomach, duodenum, adrenal glands, and the top of the urethra. Each of these organs supports a different emotion, so you may say that your midriff stores or embraces your emotions. Extra weight around the midriff may indicate extra protection around your emotions. Soreness in the midriff area may indicate stressed emotions or the inability to process or cleanse negative emotions.

Waist

Your waist represents the ability to be flexible, to turn easily, and to see the different angles and sides of life. It can show you how willing you are to change directions.

STOMACH (ABDOMEN)

Your abdomen houses your creativity and your "knowing" or gut reaction. When you experience problems such as stomach cramps or a buildup of extra weight on the abdomen, there is a blockage in your life. You may be feeling trapped, stuck, or unable to move in or out of a certain situation. You may not be following your inner knowing. Or it may be a time of gestating new ideas, or waiting for the "right" moment. Discomfort in the abdomen may also be caused by fear that you are unable to move out of a certain situation. Fear is causing you to deny your "self." Denial is the blockage causing the pain.

HIPS AND BUTTOCKS

Hips

Your hips and pelvic area represent balance, movement, and creativity. If you have problems in your hips, your life may be out of balance or you may be overloaded in one area (work versus play). It may also mean you are holding yourself back. And finally, your hips symbolize your relationship to your creativity or sexuality. If you have bulging hips, you may want to look at how you are failing to express your uniqueness or how you may be denying your creativity or your sexuality.

Buttocks

Your buttocks are the seat of power. When you have excess weight on the buttocks it usually means fear of your own power. The buttocks hold the power that you are afraid of or unwilling to handle. When the buttocks are out of shape, power is mishandled or loosely held. It is particularly interesting that in this culture large buttocks are more of a female problem than a male problem.

The buttocks are the center of all motion. When there is pain in the buttocks, power is blocked.

LEGS

Thighs

Your thighs represent strength and forward motion. When there is excess weight on the thighs it may mean you are holding onto the past or negative childhood memories associated with anger and rage. Very often if you cannot express anger, or you feel impotent in your anger, you may gain weight in your thighs.

Pain in your thighs is also an expression of repressed anger and feelings of powerlessness.

Knees

Your knees represent balance, flexibility, pride, and ego. Pain or injury in the knee may mean there is an imbalance in your life. Look at the way you balance play in relation to work, or see if your relationship is taking up all of your energy at the expense of everything else in your life. Being inflexible in work, play, and relationships may also manifest in knee problems. Do you feel rigid or stuck, must you hold yourself at attention (accountable and therefore guilty before the fact), or are you at ease?

Lower Legs

Your lower legs represent carrying you forward in life. When there's pain, you may be stopping yourself. When there is extra weight, you may be weighing yourself down, and holding yourself back. The belief here is that you "can't do it," therefore, you stop yourself.

Ankles

As with the wrists, your ankles represent your ability to take in and receive pleasure. They also represent your ability to move with ease and flexibility. Ankles hold and protect your feelings of vulnerability (e.g., Achilles tendon). Additionally, ankles represent how quickly and comfortably you communicate.

FEET AND TOES

Feet

Your feet are your base, your roots. They represent understanding yourself and others. Pain in the feet is a great limiter and reflects a fear of going forward with freedom. Feet represent caring and taking time for yourself. In addition, they also represent following your own dreams. If you have pain in your feet, look to see where you are not nurturing yourself.

Toes represent the minor details of the future.

The Big Toe represents your personal will and whether you follow through with all the minor details to carry out your will, or if you let them go unnoticed or unfulfilled.

The Second Toe represents your ambition, your skill at handling money and projects (business), your leadership ability, and your willingness to follow your intuition.

The Middle Toe represents your sense of right and wrong, your integrity with yourself and others, your search for inner truth, introspection, and your standards for behavior in the world.

The Fourth Toe represents your creative power, self-expression, and your ability to merge with others or to remain autonomous.

The Little Toe represents communication and relationships.

OTHERS

Cellulite

Cellulite represents stored anger. The body acts as a storage tank for unexpressed anger, rage, disappointment, and unhappiness. Cellulite also is a sign of self-denial and self-punishment. Somewhere, probably in childhood and then reinforced in relationships, you developed the belief that you are "wrong" and you therefore need to be punished.

Bones

Your bones represent structure. When you have bone problems you may feel rebellious against the structure of society, your home life, or the way you have structured your life. Your life may be off track, so you "stop" yourself by breaking or bruising a bone.

Fat

Fat represents fear. It is the body's way of protecting itself. Fat also can represent denial or fear of one's own feelings. The more overweight one becomes, the deeper the feelings are buried. Fat also may be a mechanism for covering over anger and disappointment.

Skin

Your skin protects your individuality. Problems with your skin show a lack of belief in your own individuality or indicate you may feel invaded by others. Your skin is a sensor. You may be denying your senses when you have skin problems, not allowing yourself to fully hear, see, feel, taste, or smell. Sensing also means allowing yourself to "sense" out situations. Skin problems may be the manifestation of your inability or unwillingness to follow your own sense of knowing.

Muscles

Your muscles hold the whole structure of your life together. They allow you to move within your structure. When muscles are sore it may mean you are having difficulty moving within the structure of your life, your life may be too structured, or you may not have enough structure.

SPECIFIC PROBLEMS

Flexibility

The word flexibility is self-explanatory. Depending on which part of your body is inflexible, you reflect the way you are in relation to the world. The limitations of each of the major body areas is exacerbated by inflexibility; for example, tightness in the back of your legs may inhibit your going forward in your life. Tightness in the chest muscles may inhibit the expression of giving or receiving love. Tightness in the lower back may cause you to be locked into fear and almost always results in pain.

Pain

Pain is an indication of self-punishment. Self-punishment always comes from guilt. Guilt can stem from any cause, any childhood belief, or as a result of paying too much attention to your critical voice. Pain can be relieved as you release your feelings of guilt.

Stiffness

Stiffness represents rigidity. It can manifest in simple muscle inflexibility or in sore and tight muscles. Spasms may result from extreme rigidity and stiff or tight thinking. When you are unwilling to be flexible with ideas and beliefs, the body may become stiff, sore, and in extreme cases, spasms may occur.

Spasms

Spasms represent tightening your thoughts through fear. When you are afraid to move forward, or afraid of the consequences, or just afraid, the muscles may spasm. Look at the area in your body that is experiencing the spasm and see if your fear is related to whatever that part of the body represents.

What is your body telling you? This book will help you to discover your own hidden subconscious beliefs, and then show you how to heal your life while creating the body you want.

Affirmation

*I am willing to allow
my body to be my teacher.
My body tells me what I need to know
about myself and my life.*

4

THE WAY YOU FEEL ABOUT YOUR BODY

"Beauty is how you feel inside,
and it reflects in your eyes.
It is not something physical."
— *Sophia Loren*

Now that you are aware of the judgmental little voice, the mind chatter, it is time to perform a head-to-toe evaluation. This evaluation will help you see how mind chatter affects your body and your self-esteem. You will begin to understand that mind chatter is not true, even though it may seem to be true at the time. It is important to realize that just as your mind can tear you apart mercilessly, it can also build you up and make you feel good. You can choose how you want to treat yourself.

In this exercise, I have written a statement for every body part. Make each statement about your body to yourself in the mirror. As you look at yourself and say positive, loving statements about your body, your mind is likely to argue. We call those arguments "responses." Write down your responses, repeat the statement, and write down any other negative thoughts. Continue to repeat the statement and write your responses until you run out of responses. Then, move on to the next body part. Do not bother to argue with your mind chatter. It is pointless, anyway. Just listen to what you say to yourself. Awareness is the key to change.

This exercise may seem difficult at times. It can be traumatic for some people; for others it is a piece of cake. If you cannot get through the whole thing, do not berate yourself. Just acknowledge yourself for every body part you can look at. Do not worry about the parts you cannot look at.

EXERCISE: *Head-to-Toe Evaluation*

Take off your clothes and stand before a full length mirror. Wait! Come back! If it is difficult for you to stand in front of a full-length mirror naked (my sister Joan tells me that she never looked in a mirror below her nose for years), do this exercise any way you can. If you cannot look in the mirror even dressed, it is okay; write how you feel about your body parts anyway (without looking).

Example:
Look at your face. Say out loud: *"I have a beautiful face."*
Write your response: *"Except for the bags under my eyes!"*
Repeat: *"I have a beautiful face."*
Write your response: *"Sure, look at the lines around your mouth. Soon you'll be needing plastic surgery!"*
Repeat: *"I have a beautiful face."*
Response: *"Except for the zit on the front of your chin."*
Continue until you run out of responses.

YOUR TURN
FACE: Say, *"I have a beautiful face."*
Write your response:_____
Say again, *"I have a beautiful face."*
Response:

1.
_____

2.
_____

3.
_____

EYES: *"I have beautiful eyes."*
Response:

1.
_____

2.
_____

3.
_____

NOSE: *"I have a great nose."*
Response:

1. _____

2. _____

3. _____

MOUTH: *"I have a beautiful mouth."*
Response:

1. _____

2. _____

3. _____

CHEEKS: *"My cheeks are beautiful/handsome."*
Response:

1. _____

2. _____

3. _____

_____

CHIN: *"My chin pleases me."*
Response:

1. _____

2. _____

3. _____

_____

EARS: *"My ears are perfect."*
Response:

1. _____

2. _____

3. _____

_____

HAIR: *"My hair is beautiful."*
Response:

1. _____

2. _____

3. _____

NECK: *"I have a beautiful neck."*
Response:

1. _____

2. _____

3. _____

SHOULDERS: *"I have lovely/strong shoulders."*
Response:

1. _____

2. _____

3. _____

UPPER ARMS: *"My upper arms are exactly the way I want them to be."*
Response:

1. _____

2. _____

3. _____

ELBOWS: *"I have great elbows."*
Response:

1. _____

2. _____

3. _____

LOWER ARMS: *"My lower arms are perfect."*
Response:

1. _____

2. _____

3. _____

WRISTS: *"My wrists are beautiful."*
Response:

1. _____

2. _____

3. _____

HANDS: *"My hands are lovely/strong/shapely."*
Response:

1. _____

2. _____

3. _____

_____

FINGERS: *"I have great shapely fingers. They are strong and flexible."*
Response:

1. _____

2. _____

3. _____

_____

UPPER BACK: *"I have a strong/beautiful upper back."*
Response:

1. _____

2. _____

3. _____

_____

MIDDLE BACK: *"I have a strong/beautiful middle back."*
Response:

1. _____

2. _____

3. _____

LOWER BACK: *"I have a strong/beautiful lower back."*
Response:

1. _____

2. _____

3. _____

CHEST: *"I have a strong/beautiful/shapely chest."*
Response:

1. _____

2. _____

3. _____

_____

BREASTS: *"I have beautiful breasts."*
Response:

1. _____

2. _____

3. _____

_____

MIDRIFF: *"My midriff is exactly the way I want it to be."*
Response:

1. _____

2. _____

3. _____

_____

WAIST: *"My waist is perfect."*
Response:

1. _____

2. _____

3. _____

STOMACH: *"I have a beautiful stomach."*
Response:

1. _____

2. _____

3. _____

HIPS: *"My hips are great."*
Response:

1. _____

2. _____

3. _____

_____

BUTTOCKS: *"I love my buttocks."*
Response:

1. _____

2. _____

3. _____

_____

THIGHS: *"I have fabulous thighs."*
Response:

1. _____

2. _____

3. _____

_____

KNEES: *"I have beautiful knees."*
Response:

1. _____

2. _____

3. _____

CALVES: *"I have strong/lovely calves."*
Response:

1. _____

2. _____

3. _____

ANKLES: *"I have great ankles."*
Response:

1. _____

2. _____

3. _____

_____

FEET: *"I love my feet."*
Response:

1. _____

2. _____

3. _____

_____

TOES: *"My toes are perfect."*
Response:

1. _____

2. _____

3. _____

_____

SKIN: *"I have beautiful skin."*
Response:

1. _____

2. _____

3. _____

   What did you learn about yourself while doing this exercise? Can you see how mind chatter (your critical voice) works? Do you see that mind chatter is merely thoughts and that your mind has made them up?

   Awareness is the first step to change. Whenever you become aware of your mind chatter, make a note of it; make a note of what is said and the circumstances that triggered it. Sometimes you can see that your mind chatter is ridiculous. Other times, mind chatter appears to be valid. Once you hear it and recognize it for what it is, you can turn it around. You do not have to be a victim of your own thoughts.

Affirmation

*I choose to be aware of my thoughts about
my body and my life.*

5

YOUR MIND AT WORK

"There is so much good in the worst of us."
— *Edward Wallace Hoch*

You are now becoming aware of how much your negative mind has been in control of your thoughts and your life. I know that these exercises are challenging, because I have done them and taught them in my classes and workshops. But they help you take a realistic look at your life, so you can decide how you want to change it. Once you decide to change, make a commitment to follow through. A commitment is a pledge or a promise that you make to yourself. This means to honor your word by sticking to it. After you take an honest look at what you want to do, start with little commitments and baby steps, so you can easily live up to your own expectations. Commitment is about you, not about other people.

As an example, this year I made a commitment to myself. I had been drinking coffee since I was sixteen years old, and diet cola for twenty-six years. Also, I had been using a substitute sweetener for as long as I can remember. When I returned from a holiday in Maui, I came down with the worst case of flu I have ever experienced. Five days of a 104 degree temperature, and stomach and head pains that were unbearable. During this time I did not drink coffee, diet cola, or use any substitute sweetener. When I finally recovered, I had already gone through five days of caffeine withdrawal during my illness, so I decided to eliminate coffee, diet cola, and substitute sweeteners from my diet altogether. I was committed.

"Finally, all my addictions are gone," I thought. Then reality struck. It was too much for me. Rebellion set in. I found myself in my old patterns. I ate ice cream that had been sitting in the freezer for months; cookies I kept for company soon followed, along with chocolates I found in the cabinet. I began to worry that I was heading toward my old eating disorder behavior. I realized that I had committed to do too much at one time. Giving up three things at once was causing more problems with my psyche than it was worth. I evaluated the situation and decided not to drink diet cola, but to allow myself coffee and substitute sweetener. My body and my psyche immediately breathed a sigh of relief and accepted this decision with comfort and renewed commitment. Now it has not been difficult for me to give up diet cola. I drink decaffeinated coffee, and have cut my substitute sweetener consumption in half. I am happy with my decision, find the commitment easy to handle, and have stopped my destructive rebellion. Eventually I will stop drinking coffee, but for now, diet cola is all I can handle giving up.

It is best to start out slowly, to make sure you can handle the commitments you make without causing yourself too much pain or discomfort. Then continue the commitment by periodically reevaluating what you really want. You may find it helpful to make lists or keep a journal. It is not important how you do this, just that you do it.

Again, remember to notice your critical voice, thank it for sharing, then breathe, and go back to the work at hand. It is a challenge to keep looking deep within. Your hidden thoughts may fight to stay secretly in your mind. They may suggest that instead of reading this book and doing these exercises, you spend time doing something constructive like eating, shopping, talking on the telephone, folding the laundry, or cleaning out closets. I am asking you to keep digging. It is you who you are finding out about, and you are a pretty special person.

When Erica came to my exercise studio she was deeply troubled. Her clothes were dirty and unpressed. Her body spilled out between the seams, her shoes were worn, her hair was unkempt. She did not look like the kind of woman who wanted to take an exercise class.

"I'm here because I'm tired of failing," she announced. "It's just time for a change." And she went to work.

I admired Erica. She exercised daily. She put herself on a diet. She bought new clothes. She had her hair styled. She got manicured and pedicured. But no matter what Erica did externally, she still failed in her career.

"Somehow I just never get good enough to make it," she told me one day. "Every time I think I've taken care of a problem, something else comes up to sabotage my success."

I recognized what was going on in Erica's life. She believed she was not good enough.

"Not good enough" is one of the major human limiting beliefs (if not the only major human limiting belief). Often it is the underpinning belief, even of the super achiever. Super achievers are so afraid of not being good enough that they drive themselves unmercifully to make that belief wrong (yet, they never feel good enough to acknowledge that they have made it).

For Erica, the "not good enough" belief worked the opposite way. No matter what she tried—and she was talented and devoted to her work—she was not good enough to succeed. Every time she did something positive for herself or her career, something negative, and seemingly external, came along to sabotage it.

Your mind might be saying, "people can't do anything about circumstances beyond their control," but even external circumstances are subject to the power of thought. Thought is creative. What you believe to be true, becomes true in your life. This means you can also attract circumstances and situations into your life that reinforce your positive subconscious beliefs about yourself. You are a very powerful person.

The good news is, you can change your life and your body simply by changing your beliefs. You can begin to change your beliefs simply by being aware of them.

Unearthing Attitudes About Yourself and Others

Sometimes the process of unearthing attitudes takes a convoluted path, and the exercises in this chapter may appear to be one of those paths. Begin to be aware of how you observe others. Notice what you observe about them, listen to your mind chatter about their bodies, particularly what you do not like. Keep a diary or journal of how you observe and what you focus on. As I have said before, the mind does not really hear "you" or "he" or "she," it hears "I." So what you are noticing about others, particularly the negatives, can apply to yourself. The good news is, when you notice positive qualities in others, they also can apply to yourself.

When Joan and I were children we spent every Easter vacation in Florida. We had many happy hours at the beach playing in the sand and swimming in the ocean, sometimes accompanied by a woman friend of the family who baby-sat for us.

Joan and I both remember our baby-sitter criticizing the bodies of people walking by our blanket: this one was too fat, that one too skinny. "Look at the way her spine curves." "Did you ever see such ugly legs?" "If I had a body like hers I would never be seen in public, let alone in a bathing suit." Thinking back on it, I had a pretty horrid picture of the way bodies were judged, and for years I found myself afraid of being judged by others.

Why was the baby-sitter so critical of others? She was always on a diet but never kept the weight off. She always complained about her own aches and pains. She hated her body and expressed her hatred by judging others harshly.

Often the critical voice can be identified, at first, by the things it says about others. The following exercise will help you see how you feel about your own body by observing the way you view others. If you judge others harshly, you probably are not comfortable with your own body. Notice the qualities or body parts you criticize most about others. You may have a problem with those qualities in yourself or those areas of your body.

I am very conscious of other women's stomachs, buttocks, and thighs. I am very conscious of my own stomach, buttocks, and thighs. I do not spend much time watching other women's hips or breasts, but then, I love my own. I notice arms, but only because I think mine are beautiful. It goes like that. You may be surprised by how you transfer your own judgment of yourself to others. The wonderful thing about this exercise is that once you locate your judgment areas, you can take a more realistic look at yourself and your own body. Then you can begin to change your negative feelings.

EXERCISE: *Observing Others, Observing Yourself*

There are two parts to this exercise. The first part is to observe yourself observing. All day long, as you walk down the street, as you drive your car or ride on public transportation, as you work and play, be aware of your thoughts about other people—the way they act, the way they look. At the end of the day, or more often if it's possible, write down those thoughts and observations in a diary.

Your diary might look something like this:
"I noticed that I'm always focusing on people's stomachs. Today I saw a man who looked pregnant, and a woman looked like she was carrying a small ball on her front. It's funny that I feel strongly about the stomach. I remember when I was in summer stock and the costume designer said that she was going to have to make adjustments to all the costumes to cover up for my stomach. Oh my, this has to be an area I think about a lot.

"I notice that I'm being pretty negative about all bodies in general. I don't seem to see a lot of beauty in the human body at all. I think there's a correlation between what I see and the fact that I'm not too pleased with any part of myself.

"Today, I have seen nothing but beautiful people. People with slender thighs, trim ankles and the kinds of knees that look good in fashion magazines. I think the human body is a celebration of beauty and I'm delighted to be human."

The second half of this exercise is to practice not making yourself wrong for what you notice and how you feel. Your critical voice or mind chatter is not right. Become aware of your reactions to your mind chatter. Your thoughts may scold you for being late: "You're late, you're always late." "Can't you get anywhere on time?" "You're getting a reputation for always being late." "You were always late as a child and it made everyone angry." "Aren't you ever going to grow up?" Scolding yourself for being late does not make you be on time. In fact, the more you focus on always being late the more likely you are to continue to always be late. Take the pressure off yourself. Change the focus from being late, to getting where you are going at exactly the right time. Tell yourself you have plenty of time to get where you want to go.

As you become more aware of your negative thoughts and learn to control your mind chatter, your life and your body will begin to change. Each step along the way of understanding yourself takes you a little closer to creating the life and the body that will make you happy.

Affirmation

I see the positive qualities of life and people.
I see the positive aspects of myself.

6

HOW YOUR THOUGHTS SABOTAGE YOUR SUCCESS

*"My meaningless thoughts create
my meaningless world."*
— *The Course in Miracles*

Many of us refuse, or as I say, deflect compliments. Since we only hear what we really believe to be true, it may be difficult to acknowledge nice things about ourselves and this can keep us from creating the lives and the bodies that we want.

Several of my clients had self-limiting belief systems. Charlotte believed that other people would always react negatively to her as an overweight woman. Even when others did not react as negatively as she thought they would, she still did not try to do some things, assuming that her being overweight would eventually cause her to fail. Mary wanted to be a model but gave up the idea because she was self-conscious about chicken pox scars that she had on her face. But Beth, who believed she had neither a beautiful face nor a gorgeous body, became a photographer's model for her extraordinary hands.

The following exercises will help you define the challenges (some people call them problems) that you need to face with your body and in your life. Once they are defined, you can more easily overcome your challenges.

EXERCISE: *Defining Your Challenges—Part I*

A. The challenges I have with my body interfere with my ability to achieve success because:

Example:
People don't take me seriously as an exercise expert. How can an expert be trusted if she has too much fat on her arms, her stomach, and her buttocks?

YOUR TURN

_____

_____

_____

_____

B. How the challenges I have with my body serve me:

Example:
My arms remind me to continue to exercise. Without them as a reminder, I tend to let exercise go.

YOUR TURN

_____

_____

_____

_____

C. Another way the challenges I have with my body serve me:

Example:
My arms continually remind me to affirm my willingness to embrace life fully and with joy, to allow myself to fly.

YOUR TURN

_____

_____

_____

_____

D. *Another way the challenges I have with my body serve me:*

Example:
They keep me from getting to the top. People notice my arms and therefore discount what I have to say. Perhaps I'm afraid of getting to the top.

YOUR TURN

_____

_____

_____

_____

E. *Choose other challenges and keep going.*

_____

_____

_____

_____

_____

_____

_____

_____

_____

_____

_____

_____

_____

_____

_____

EXERCISE: *Defining Your Challenges — Part II*

A. *The area of my body, or body challenge, I have now identified as limiting:*

Example:
My upper arms are the worst offenders.

YOUR TURN

_____

_____

_____

_____

B. *Five ways I use this area of my body, or body challenge, to create limits to my success are:*

Example:
1. I hold myself back because I believe people won't take me seriously.
2. I feel insecure about my looks because of my "fat" arms.
3. I put myself down because I believe I ought to be able to do something about it.
4. I don't take in all of what's offered to me in my life.
5. I hold myself back so that I don't intimidate others (especially if I'm in a relationship).

YOUR TURN

1. _____

2. _____

3. _____

4. _____

5. _____

C. *Five negative things I say to myself, or to others, to deflect a compliment are:*

Example:
1. *Thank you, but I really need to get my arms in shape.*
2. *And you look beautiful, too.*
3. *You ought to see me when I'm rested.*
4. *I just got my hair done.*
5. *Thanks, another 10 pounds and I'll look great.*

YOUR TURN

1. _____

2. _____

3. _____

4. _____

5. _____

D. *Five ways I put myself down before others can do it, are:*

Example:
1. *I'd be in great shape if I weren't carrying these extra 10 pounds. (I'm too fat.)*
2. *I'd better get out of this relationship before he leaves me. (I'm not good enough.)*
3. *My son would be able to handle his life better if I'd given him more direction as a child. (I'm a lousy mother. I'm incompetent.)*
4. *I eat too much, no wonder I can't lose weight. (I have no willpower.)*
5. *I'm a space cadet when it comes to following directions. (I'm stupid.)*

YOUR TURN

1. _____

2. _____

3. _____

4. _____

5. _____

E.   What are the recurring themes to your negative beliefs? For me there are several:
1. I'm too fat.
2. I'm not good enough.
3. I'm a lousy mother.
4. I'm incompetent.
5. I'm stupid.

YOUR TURN

1. _____

2. _____

3. _____

4. _____

5. _____

What you have learned about yourself while doing this exercise might surprise you. I certainly have been surprised about myself. Remember, do not be judgmental about what you have found out about yourself, your past, or your family. This exercise only serves to illustrate what you have done in the past that may be influencing your present. Now you are at a point where you can make some choices. You can choose to continue the way things are in your life, or you can change your mind.

Affirmation

My challenges are easy to overcome.
The past is over.
Now I can be whatever I choose to be.

7

CREATING A NEW PERSPECTIVE

"It's only a thought,
and a thought can be changed."

— *Louise L. Hay*

Y ou can change your reality, but first you must change your thoughts. There are many tools for changing thoughts; to begin, simply become aware of them. By understanding the underlying thoughts that limit your life, you can start to create your new life.

The way we see our lives today is based on our perceptions of the past. Our beliefs are based on the way we have seen things since we were children. As we change our childhood viewpoint, we can create a new adult. My friend Sharon said to me one day as I was railing against my mother, "Someone else could have experienced the same episode and drawn completely different conclusions. Your mother is innocent. She did the best she could with the information and the experience she had. It is the conclusions you drew from her behavior that are upsetting you."

The problem with blame and guilt is that they do not change anything. Blaming does not make anything better. In fact, if you really want to feel lousy, get into a heavy session with an agreeable friend and talk about all the things that others have done to you over the years. It's true, things do happen, but you don't have to dwell on them and keep them alive today in the present.

Let us for a moment look at a chapter from my youth. Bonnie, my mother, was one of the top rock climbers in the world. She and my father, Dick, thought there was no healthier way to spend a weekend than hanging by their fingertips a thousand feet up in the air admiring the view. I loved to rock climb; from my earliest moments I could think of no better afternoon activity, with the possible exception of horseback riding. My sister, Joan, on the other hand, considered these weekend activities to be a plot against all that was enjoyable. Joan's idea of a fun way to spend a Saturday was in bed with a good book and a snack.

Innocently, by taking us rock climbing, Bonnie thought she was promoting our health and strength and sharing a wonderful activity with us. For me, it was true. I have delightful memories of achievement and evenings around the campfire, while Joan has miserable memories of fear, ridicule, and discomfort. We climbed the same cliffs, very often at the same time, but our experiences and conclusions were totally different.

Since Joan reached puberty she has been severely overweight. Once, when we were discussing rock climbing, Joan talked about the problem she had telling Bonnie how much she disliked this kind of activity. It wasn't just rock climbing, it was downhill skiing and horseback riding competition, too. Bonnie was an avid sports competitor and expected her daughters not only to follow suit but to enjoy themselves, too.

Joan told me that she sees how her being overweight served her. It gave her the power to say "no" to mother's sports activities without running the risk of actually saying "no." It stands to reason that if you weigh 150-200 pounds, no one is going to make you ride a horse in a race. It stands to reason that if you are too heavy to pull yourself up the face of a cliff, no one is going to want to haul you up. Fat represents power and safety to Joan.

She can choose to spend her life blaming Bonnie for subjecting her to what Bonnie thought was pleasurable. Or, she can look at it, acknowledge that they didn't agree on what constituted an idea of pleasure, know that it was not done on purpose to make her miserable, and let it go. Joan's much happier when she does that. Still, her subconscious decision that fat and power are companions frequently gets in her way. This is how a negative and a positive get confused. Any time Joan gets herself into a situation where she feels powerless, she gains weight. I can always tell how she feels in her life by whether she's gaining or losing.

Joan learned that she could never lose her fat as long as it represented her power and safety. Only when she believed she could say "no, thank you" any time she didn't want to do something, could she begin working on her body. She is finding power in herself rather than in her excess weight.

Another example of subconscious choice is shown by Catherine, one of my clients. She came to my studio several years ago because she wanted to correct her posture. Catherine had rounded shoulders, a caved-in chest, and her lower spine was flat, which caused pain in her lower back. She moved like the invisible woman, and was the most unmemorable woman I have ever met. I cannot even recall what she looked like, only that I worked with her. Catherine seemed so uncomfortable in her body that she did not want anyone to notice she even had a body. Only a painful back problem kept Catherine from ignoring her body completely.

I placed Catherine in a regular exercise class, with special exercises to strengthen her back and shoulders as well as to stretch her pectorals. But that was only part of the program. She also started learning how to figure out why she created the physical problems in the first place.

Catherine had no idea that an experience, a thought, or a belief, could have anything to do with her body. She believed she was weak and inflexible, with poor posture habits, and she blamed herself for being sloppy. It took months for Catherine to discover that at a very early age she decided to disappear, partly because of how she felt about her mother's personality, and partly because of a childhood experience, which made her terrified of men.

At the time Catherine was nearing puberty, her mother, then divorced, had a boyfriend who would play with Catherine, creating wrestling matches and tickle-fights. He would touch her body and make sexual remarks and jokes about her increasing sexuality. The boyfriend's inappropriate sexual behavior represented a double threat to Catherine. She was afraid her mother might think she was competing for the man's attentions, and she believed that her mother would become enraged with the man if Catherine expressed how terrified she had become of him. Any way she looked at it, Catherine felt she couldn't win, so she got as small as possible. In effect, she mutilated her body by twisting it inward, so that she would seem unattractive. She disappeared.

Eventually, the mother caught on to her boyfriend's mistreatment of her daughter and he was asked to leave. But Catherine's problem didn't leave. She carried it into her adult life, never realizing where it originated.

As we looked at Catherine's childhood and her beliefs, we began to discover Catherine's adult beliefs about men and sexuality. As long as she stayed invisible, there was no possibility that she would deal with her fear of sexuality. What Catherine had to do was create a belief that she was safe. So as she continued with the physical exercises, I suggested that she see a counselor who specialized in sexual abuse.

Catherine's posture improved because she was willing to dig deep enough to find out why she decided to create bad posture and a weak, inflexible body. When she learned how her bad posture actually protected her, she was able to begin to change her unconscious beliefs through counseling, affirmations, visualizations, and the other exercises outlined in this book. While she changed the muscle structure of her body, she eliminated the need to maintain her bad posture in order to feel safe.

Catherine has made a great deal of headway. She walks freely. She has changed her hair and her clothing. Her shoulders are straight, her chest is no longer caved in. She has greater lung capacity because she has opened her chest. This has resulted in more oxygen in her system and more energy overall.

What we learn from Catherine and Joan is that people make certain decisions about their lives based on experiences beginning from childhood. These decisions are stored in the subconscious and are out-pictured by the body in the form of posture, health, the way we carry weight, and the way we look and act. These beliefs may look negative, but on a subconscious level they are positive for us. The problem is, the subconscious will continue to believe they are positive long after they no longer work to protect us or serve our needs. When that happens, it is vital to identify the belief, change it, and move forward with your life.

In order to reprogram your subconscious, it is important to reframe your negative beliefs. One way to do that is with "turnarounds," taking the old, negative belief and turning it around to make it positive. At first it may seem ridiculous, but you will find that it works, it is fun, and your beliefs really do change. Then, as your beliefs change, so does your life, and your body.

EXERCISE: *Positive Turnarounds*

List all of the negative statements that you have made about yourself in Chapter Six and turn them into positive statements.

Example:
Negative Statement
I'd be in great shape if I weren't carrying these extra ten pounds.

Positive Turnaround
My weight is right for me at this time in my life. I'm in perfect shape.

Negative Statement
I had better get out of this relationship before he leaves me. (I'm not good enough.)

Positive Turnaround
I am loved for who I am.

Negative Statement
My son would be able to handle his life better if I'd given him more direction as a child. (I'm a lousy mother. I'm incompetent.)

Positive Turnaround
I am the perfect mother. I did the best I could with the information I had at the time.

Negative Statement
I'm a space cadet when it comes to following directions. (I'm stupid.)

Positive Turnaround
Even the most complex directions are easy to follow.

YOUR TURN

Negative Statement

_____

_____

Positive Turnaround

_____

_____

Negative Statement

_____

_____

Positive Turnaround

_____

_____

Negative Statement

_____

_____

Positive Turnaround

_____

_____

Negative Statement

_____

_____

Positive Turnaround

_____

_____

Negative Statement

_____

_____

Positive Turnaround

_____

_____

You may be amazed at how much easier it is to think of negatives than it is to think of positives. That is early childhood training. But just as we had to learn to find our faults and think negatively, we can learn to think positively. Fortunately, as you begin to train your mind to think positively it will become easier and easier.

Take a look at your underlying beliefs, the ones that form the foundations for all your negative thoughts about yourself. Start with the ones that rule the negative statements you have just made about yourself in the previous exercise. It is very important to turn around these underlying beliefs because they color your entire reality about yourself. List them and then write your positive turn-around beneath them. You may want to make extra copies of your new turn-around beliefs and put them up in various places in your house. The bathroom mirror is an excellent location. Just think! First thing every morning you will see a positive belief about yourself.

EXERCISE: *Challenging Your Underlying Beliefs*

Old Underlying Belief
I'm too fat.

Positive Turnaround
I'm the perfect size.

Old Underlying Belief
I'm stupid.

Positive Turnaround
I'm extremely intelligent.

Old Underlying Belief
I'm not good enough.

Positive Turnaround
I'm perfect just the way I am.

YOUR TURN

Old Underlying Belief

_____

_____

Positive Turnaround

_____

_____

Old Underlying Belief

_____

_____

Positive Turnaround

_____

_____

Old Underlying Belief

_____

_____

Positive Turnaround

_____

_____

Old Underlying Belief

_____

_____

Positive Turnaround

_____

_____

Old Underlying Belief

_____

_____

Positive Turnaround

_____

_____

Make it a point to take any negative thought that you hear your mind throw at you and automatically rephrase it as a positive. This takes practice. For example, let's go back to how you can "beat yourself up" if you're late. Your mind starts to scream at you, "You're late, you're always late! Can't you get anywhere on time?" Consciously change it to "I have all the time I need to get where I have to go or do what I need to do." Another example, and one I use often is, "How will I pay the bills? I don't have enough money!" Change this to "All my needs are met in present time." Eventually your subconscious will get bored with being corrected and the negatives will begin to slow down. (The good news for me is that all my needs are met in present time and, now that I know it, I can stop yelling at myself in the first place. I'm still working on lateness.)

When you begin to root out your underlying beliefs and reframe them, your self-worth and self-esteem will soar. What seemed difficult will become easy; you will enjoy your body and your life more.

Ultimately, you are working toward long periods of time when you hear no mind chatter. For the moment, it's good enough just to hear positive chatter.

Affirmation

My challenges are easy to overcome.
The past is over.
Now I can be whatever I choose to be.

8

GOAL SETTING

"Plan your work, work your plan."
— *Tom Watson, IBM*

Not many people make plans, set goals, or write down the things that they want to accomplish in their lives. Yet these can be the most powerful stepping stones toward achieving what we want.

There was an interesting study conducted at Yale University in 1953. That year's graduating seniors were asked a number of questions, one of which was, "Have you set clear, specific goals for your life and have you written down your plans to accomplish them?" Only 3 percent of the graduating class said that they had written down their specific goals and plans. Twenty years later, researchers interviewed survivors of that class and found, to their astonishment, that the 3 percent who had written down their goals and plans were worth more financially than the remaining 97 percent of their classmates all put together.

I find that unless I write down my goals, I file them in the back of my mind and "sort of get them done...maybe." Worse, I focus on one goal to the exclusion of others, and then find myself in trouble because I did not pay attention to other things I needed to do.

My friend Joe, who ran a small advertising agency, loved working with established clients, but hated looking for new ones. Every six months, when he came to the end of a billing period, he would have to lay off his secretary because he did not have any new clients to keep the business going. His financial difficulty would continue for a month or two until he reestablished himself. Eventually he started working with goals that included finding new clients as he was working with existing ones, and his business began to flourish.

My life and my body work better when I work with a structured program that includes writing down what I want to accomplish. I define my goals and structure them in a way that keeps them in the front of my mind so I do not get sidetracked. As I complete each goal, I check it off my list, and congratulate myself for succeeding.

Before you can begin working with your goals to create the body and life that you want, you must decide exactly what you are going to create. Begin with a statement defining what you want. Since this book is about the body, state what you want your body to be like. For example: I want my body to be toned, strong, flexible, and healthy.

EXERCISE: *The Way I Want My Body to Be*

Complete the following thought—
The way I want my body to be is:

Example:
I am generally happy with my body the way it is. I do want the undersides of my upper arms to be thinner and more toned. I love my hips just the way they are. I'd like my rear end to be a little smaller and tighter, and if I could flatten my stomach just a bit I'd be very happy. My breasts are perfect and my back is exceptionally beautiful, but tighter and more defined thighs would really please me.

YOUR TURN
       The way I want my body to be is:

_____

_____

_____

_____

_____

_____

Now that you have described your entire body, look at each part separately. This gives you an opportunity to focus on those parts of your body that you would like to change. Remember, be gentle with yourself. Just write down your various body parts and describe how you would like them to be.

Example:
I want my upper arms to be: Firm, toned, well-defined, strong, and feminine.

YOUR TURN

I want my _____ *to be:*

_____

_____

I want my _____ *to be:*

_____

_____

I want my _____ *to be:*

_____

_____

I want my _____ *to be:*

_____

_____

I want my _____ *to be:*

_____

_____

I want my _____ *to be:*

_____

_____

_____

I want my _____ *to be:*

_____

_____

I want my _____ *to be:*

_____

_____

I want my _____ *to be:*

_____

_____

I want my _____ *to be:*

_____

_____

Next, create a picture of exactly what you want. To do this, use a method called treasure mapping.

Treasure Mapping

Treasure mapping is a fun and creative way of picturing things the way you want them to be. A treasure map is a collage (a cut and paste picture) of whatever you want: money, an ideal body, a home, a car, vacations, jewelry, a relationship, a family. It is made by cutting pictures, words, and phrases from magazines or newspapers, and pasting them on a piece of paper to create a picture that has meaning for you. It is fun. Buy sheets of letters at an art or stationery store and write special words and phrases. SPLENDIFEROUS is one I really like.

Make treasure maps for every facet of your life. It is a wonderful way to spend an afternoon, and it gives you concentrated time to create a picture of what you want. I make my treasure maps on a huge poster board; my sister Joan likes to put hers on the inside of a file folder so it will stand up by itself, and so she can fold it away when people come to visit. Most people do not share their treasure maps with others but place them in a location where they can see it at least once a day.

There are several things you need to include in your treasure map. One is you. If you are working on a treasure map of your ideal body, your head could be put on top of bodies that look the way you want to look in different poses or while involved in your favorite activities. If you do not have photographs of yourself to use, ask a friend to take some, cut off the body, and paste your head on pictures you like.

Your treasure map also might have something in it that represents a deity or higher power to you. It does not have to be a conventional picture of Christ on the cross. As they say in Alcoholics Anonymous, if you cannot see your higher power as God, see it as anything you choose. One of my clients, Ellen, found some wonderful pictures of South American primitive drawings in an art book. She photocopied them to use as her deity. Alice, another client, found herself visualizing the woman at the beginning of the Columbia Pictures movies. My mother, Bonnie, calls herself a druid and uses pictures of trees. Use whatever represents a power greater than yourself that you can enlist to help you get what you want.

Your treasure map might also contain a sentence similar to the following:

"This or something better now manifests in my life with good to all concerned."

How Treasure Mapping Reveals Your Hidden Agendas

My client, Alex, said she wanted to weigh 120 pounds, but she kept losing and gaining and losing and gaining. One day as she was making a treasure map, she discovered something remarkable. She was positively repulsed by the models in magazines. She did not want her head attached to any of those stringy, skinny bodies. She liked "people of substance." She was attracted to heavy men and she was comfortable with heavy women. She did not want to weigh 120 pounds, after all; she wanted to lose just enough weight to be comfortable.

Making a treasure map while you are goal-setting helps you create a visual image of what you want. This process is powerful. Be specific about details if you can. Be sure you are asking for exactly what you really want. Then, after you truly desire it, you must sincerely believe that you can have it. Combine desire with belief and you will get it.

I had a friend who made a complete life plan treasure map and pasted a baby into the picture. Soon afterward she became pregnant. Unfortunately, she had not pasted in a husband to be the father of her baby. She had not yet attracted the man she wanted to be with forever, the house they would live in, or the money to support the child. I have learned to be very careful to ask for only the things I am ready to have.

Treasure mapping can also show you what you are not ready to have. One year I decided to do a treasure map on relationships, but my mind did not want to deal with relationships, so I could not find one romantic scene in a magazine. Instead, I saw only living spaces. I would think, "Now wait a minute, I want to look at loving people," and my eyes would pick out the perfect sofa. Obviously, I was not ready for a relationship at that moment, indeed, shortly thereafter, I moved into an exceptionally beautiful new home. It is a perfect home for one person and I am very happy to live alone.

Next, define some goals to help you achieve the things you want to do with your body.

For some people, changing the way they eat would allow them to lose ten pounds in twelve weeks. That is a good goal. Begin with only a few goals that address things you want to achieve for your body. Be sure the goals are possible. It is self-defeating to say that you will exercise every day when, realistically, you will end up exercising only once or twice a week, feel guilty for not keeping your commitment, and then stop entirely. Start slowly. Proceed one step at a time.

EXERCISE: *Goal Setting*

Finish the following sentence.
A goal I could achieve that would be nice for my body is:

Example:
1. Exercising to the MetaFitness Video twice a week.
2. Visit the gym and work out on Nautilus equipment to tighten the muscles under my upper arms.
3. Horseback ride once a week.
4. Have a massage once a week.

YOUR TURN

Goals I could achieve that would be nice for my body are:

1. _____

2. _____

3. _____

4. _____

5. _____

6. _____

Setting Tasks

After defining your broad goals, think about what tasks you need to perform in order to complete these goals.

EXERCISE: *Setting Tasks*

What do your tasks look like?
Five tasks that support my goals this week are:

Example:
1. Investigating exercise clubs in my new neighborhood and becoming a member.
2. Calling riding stables or borrowing my friend Christine's horse.
3. Calling the masseuse to set up a series of appointments and paying for them ahead of time to be sure I commit myself.
4. Making sure I exercise early in the morning before I get caught up in my day.
5. Getting a friend to exercise with me so I will have more fun.

YOUR TURN

Tasks that support my goals this week are:

1. _____

_____

2. _____

_____

3. _____

_____

4. _____

_____

5. _____

_____

When I first learned to plan and set goals, I could only see to the end of the week. After awhile I could see two weeks ahead, but looking ten weeks ahead was very difficult, and if you asked me about next year, I would freeze up and not be able to think at all. Planning takes learning. Once you are able to set goals and tasks one week ahead, try to look forward two weeks, then three, then four, then eight. Do not get upset with yourself if setting goals is difficult in the beginning. It gets easier.

Affirmation

I am able to clearly see what I want
and plan a way to get it.

9

WORKING WITH GOALS AND TASKS

"I have learned to use the word
'impossible' with the greatest caution."
— *Wernher von Braun*

*E*very Monday, I review what I did the previous week. I measure what percentage of my stated goals and tasks I completed, and I write down any goals and tasks I completed in addition to those originally planned. Then I take time out to acknowledge myself for my accomplishments. On another sheet of paper, I write down my goals for the upcoming week and the tasks I need to do to accomplish them.

I also look at what happened last week, what I did not do, and what consistently is not getting done. I do not make myself wrong for it, I just check to see whether I have set a goal I really do not want at this time. If that is the case, I usually drop it or I put it on the back burner until I'm more prepared to face it. Or if it absolutely requires my attention, I work on it with all my affirmations and visualizations to make certain it gets the extra push it needs. (We will discuss these techniques in Chapter Ten.)

A client of mine, Edna, put down dieting as her goal, but she steadily gained weight. Under normal circumstances we would have just let her gain, but Edna was having physical problems: her legs, her back, and her feet were suffering from her weight problem. This was not a time to let Edna's resistance be in charge. We brought the whole MetaFitness program to bear on Edna's life and what she discovered was that her inner voice told her to go on a fast, but she was afraid to do so. She tried everything else, instead of fasting as her subconscious kept telling her to do. And everything else did not work.

When Edna finally went on a fast, she began to lose weight. But more importantly, because she began to detoxify her system, which is what her subconscious knew she had to do, the pain in her body began to go away. Her feet stopped hurting, as did her legs and back. She began to feel healthy for the first time in years. Once she finished the fast and her body began to feel better, she developed goals and a program for keeping her body healthy and her weight stable.

Remember, your body took time to get the way it is; it will take time to reshape it. Make it easy on yourself by taking one step at a time.

The following goals, tasks, and acknowledgements are to be filled out every week for twelve weeks.

EXERCISE: *Goals, Tasks, and Acknowledgements*

Date   Week 1

Goals

I wish to achieve the following goals this week:

Example:
1. Make appointments with myself to do the writing required to meet my deadline.
2. Take time daily for outdoor exercise such as walking or hiking.
3. Monitor my consumption of coffee and substitute sweeteners.

YOUR TURN

1. _____

2. _____

3. _____

4. _____

5. _____

6. _____

Tasks

I wish to complete the following tasks that support my goals this week:

Example:
1. Make sure I have enough computer floppy disks.
2. Turn my answering machine on while I work to ensure that I DON'T answer the phone.
3. Purchase more decaffeinated coffee.
4. Call my friend Toni to arrange for an afternoon hike.

YOUR TURN

1. _____

_____

2. _____

_____

3. _____

_____

4. _____

_____

5. _____

_____

6. _____

_____

Acknowledgements

I wish to acknowledge myself for the following goals and tasks that I wrote down this week:

Example:
1. When the telephone rang I let the answering machine pick up the calls and I didn't even monitor them.

2. I worked steadily at the computer all morning, writing enough pages to stay on schedule to meet my deadline.
3. When I went shopping in the afternoon, I picked up extra computer floppy disks and decaffeinated coffee.
4. I used only half my usual amount of substitute sweetener in my coffee all day.
5. I went for a walk in the mountains with my friend Toni.

YOUR TURN

1. _____

_____

2. _____

_____

3. _____

_____

4. _____

_____

5. _____

_____

6. _____

_____

Bonus Acknowledgements

I wish to acknowledge myself for the following goals that I did not write down at the beginning of the week:

Example:
1. I spoke with my agent about a new project I may be doing in the fall.
2. I prepared a large salad with all sorts of raw fresh vegetables for my lunch each day.

YOUR TURN

1. _____

2. _____

3. _____

4. _____

5. _____

6. _____

*Percentage of goals completed:*_____

> *Each Monday, make sure you look over the goals you set last week and write in what percentage you completed.*

Date   Week 2

Goals

> *I wish to achieve the following goals this week:*

1. _____

2. _____

3. _____

4. _____

5. _____

6. _____

Tasks

> *I wish to complete the following tasks that support my goals this week:*

1. _____

2. _____

3. _____

4. _____

5. _____

6. _____

Acknowledgements

I wish to acknowledge myself for the following goals and tasks that I wrote down this week:

1. _____

_____

2. _____

_____

3. _____

_____

4. _____

_____

5. _____

_____

6. _____

_____

Bonus Acknowledgements

I wish to acknowledge myself for the following goals that I did not write down at the beginning of the week:

1. _____

2. _____

3. _____

4. _____

5. _____

6. _____

*Percentage of goals completed:*_____

Date _____ Week 3

Goals

I wish to achieve the following goals this week:

1. _____

2. _____

3. _____

4. _____

5. _____

6. _____

Tasks

I wish to complete the following tasks that support my goals this week:

1. _____

_____

2 . _____

_____

3 . _____

_____

4 . _____

_____

5 . _____

_____

6 . _____

_____

Acknowledgements

I wish to acknowledge myself for the following goals and tasks that I wrote down this week:

1. _____

_____

2 . _____

_____

3 . _____

_____

4 . _____

_____

5 . _____

_____

6. _____

_____

Bonus Acknowledgements

I wish to acknowledge myself for the following goals that I did not write down at the beginning of the week:

1. _____

2. _____

3. _____

4. _____

5. _____

6. _____

*Percentage of goals completed:*_____

Date _____ **Week 4**

Goals

I wish to achieve the following goals this week:

1. _____

2. _____

3. _____

4. _____

5. _____

6. _____

Tasks

I wish to complete the following tasks that support my goals this week:

1. _____

_____

2. _____

_____

3. _____

_____

4. _____

_____

5. _____

_____

6. _____

_____

Acknowledgements

I wish to acknowledge myself for the following goals and tasks that I wrote down this week:

1. _____

_____

2. _____

_____

3. _____

_____

4.
_____

_____

5.
_____

_____

6.
_____

_____

Bonus Acknowledgements

I wish to acknowledge myself for the following goals that I did not write down at the beginning of the week:

1. _____

2. _____

3. _____

4. _____

5. _____

6. _____

*Percentage of goals completed:*_____

Date   Week 5

Goals

I wish to achieve the following goals this week:

1. _____

2. _____

3. _____

4. _____

5. _____

6. _____

Tasks

I wish to complete the following tasks that support my goals this week:

1. _____

_____

2. _____

_____

3. _____

_____

4. _____

_____

5. _____

_____

6. _____

_____

Acknowledgements

I wish to acknowledge myself for the following goals and tasks that I wrote down this week:

1. _____

_____

2. _____

_____

3. _____

_____

4. _____

_____

5. _____

_____

6. _____

_____

Bonus Acknowledgements

I wish to acknowledge myself for the following goals that I did not write down at the beginning of the week:

1. _____

2. _____

3. _____

4. _____

5. _____

6. _____

*Percentage of goals completed:*_____

Date _____ Week 8

Goals

I wish to achieve the following goals this week:

1. _____

2. _____

3. _____

4. _____

5. _____

6. _____

Tasks

I wish to complete the following tasks that support my goals this week:

1. _____

_____

2. _____

_____

3. _____

_____

4. _____

_____

5. _____

_____

6. _____

_____

Acknowledgements

I wish to acknowledge myself for the following goals and tasks that I wrote down this week:

1. _____

_____

2. _____

_____

3. _____

_____

4. _____

_____

5. _____

_____

6. _____

_____

Bonus Acknowledgements

I wish to acknowledge myself for the following goals that I did not write down at the beginning of the week:

1. _____
2. _____
3. _____
4. _____
5. _____
6. _____

*Percentage of goals completed:*_____

Date _____ Week 9

Goals

I wish to achieve the following goals this week:

1. _____
2. _____
3. _____
4. _____
5. _____
6. _____

Tasks

I wish to complete the following tasks that support my goals this week:

1. _____

_____

2. _____

_____

3. _____

_____

4. _____

_____

5. _____

_____

6. _____

_____

Acknowledgements

I wish to acknowledge myself for the following goals and tasks that I wrote down this week:

1. _____

_____

2. _____

_____

3. _____

_____

4. _____

_____

5.
_____

_____

6.
_____

_____

Bonus Acknowledgements

I wish to acknowledge myself for the following goals that I did not write down at the beginning of the week:

1. _____

2. _____

3. _____

4. _____

5. _____

6. _____

*Percentage of goals completed:*_____

Date   Week 10

Goals

I wish to achieve the following goals this week:

1. _____

2. _____

3. _____

4. _____

5. _____

6. _____

Tasks

I wish to complete the following tasks that support my goals this week:

1. _____

_____

2. _____

_____

3. _____

_____

4. _____

_____

5. _____

_____

6. _____

_____

Acknowledgements

I wish to acknowledge myself for the following goals and tasks that I wrote down this week:

1. _____

_____

2. _____

_____

3. _____

_____

4. _____

5. _____

6. _____

Bonus Acknowledgements

I wish to acknowledge myself for the following goals that I did not write down at the beginning of the week:

1. _____
2. _____
3. _____
4. _____
5. _____
6. _____

*Percentage of goals completed:*_____

Date _____ Week 11

Goals

I wish to achieve the following goals this week:

1. _____
2. _____
3. _____
4. _____
5. _____
6. _____

Tasks

I wish to complete the following tasks that support my goals this week:

1. _____

_____

2. _____

_____

3. _____

_____

4. _____

_____

5. _____

_____

6. _____

_____

Acknowledgements

I wish to acknowledge myself for the following goals and tasks that I wrote down this week:

1. _____

_____

2. _____

_____

3. _____

_____

4. _____

_____

5. _____

_____

6. _____

_____

Bonus Acknowledgements

I wish to acknowledge myself for the following goals that I did not write down at the beginning of the week:

1. _____

2. _____

3. _____

4. _____

5. _____

6. _____

*Percentage of goals completed:*_____

Date _____ **Week 12**

Goals

I wish to achieve the following goals this week:

1. _____

2. _____

3. _____

4. _____

5. _____

6. _____

Tasks

I wish to complete the following tasks that support my goals this week:

1. _____

_____

2. _____

_____

3. _____

_____

4. _____

_____

5. _____

_____

6. _____

_____

Acknowledgements

I wish to acknowledge myself for the following goals and tasks that I wrote down this week:

1. _____

_____

2. _____

_____

3. _____

_____

4. _____

_____

5. _____

_____

6. _____

_____

Bonus Acknowledgements

I wish to acknowledge myself for the following goals that I did not write down at the beginning of the week:

1. _____
2. _____
3. _____
4. _____
5. _____
6. _____

Percentage of goals completed: _____

Be sure to check back with your plan each week. I've found that working with someone else helps me to achieve these goals. (I work best with my sister, Petie. I use her as my audience for "show and tell," and having someone to check in with motivates me.) Enjoy learning to set and meet your goals. My new motto in life is, "If it isn't fun, why do it?"

HAVE FUN!

Affirmation

I easily set and achieve my goals.
Each task I complete is an accomplishment
I gladly acknowledge.

10

USING AFFIRMATIONS,
VISUALIZATIONS, AND EXERCISES

*"Whatever the mind of man
can conceive and believe, it can achieve."*
— *Napoleon Hill*

We are now about to stop digging through old negative beliefs and start building on the positive by using affirmations and visualizations. These two tools can help you to change your life and your body, to love yourself, and to get what you want.

An affirmation, in its most fundamental form, is anything you think or say. There are positive affirmations and negative affirmations. Your positive thoughts and speech help you enhance your life and change negative beliefs. Negative phrases, and sometimes whole stories that you repeat, reinforce the aspects of your life or your body that make you unhappy. By repeating positive affirmations over and over in your thoughts and your speech, you can change your negative subconscious beliefs.

Where You Are Coming From

While teaching exercise classes for the past twenty years, I have observed that many people use negative affirmations throughout class. They will say,

"Look at my hips." "Oh no, cellulite." "My stomach is still too fat." "My arms are so ugly." "God, I hate exercising, isn't there an easier way?" They affirm that they hate exercise, then their bodies and their lives do not change. A high percentage of these people either drop out of exercise programs or they injure themselves as a subconscious excuse to get out of a class. They know the class is good for them, but their negative affirmations rule their minds and their bodies.

My friend Louise L. Hay, a metaphysical counselor, and I were having tea one day after I had just moved into my new home in the country. I felt a little isolated and uncertain about my social life, and I said, "Looks like there won't be any men in my life this year." In her inimitable way, Louise calmly said, "I wouldn't affirm that if I were you." I understood immediately.

Begin to watch what you say. Make sure you speak positively, and your life can become a completely positive experience. Silva Mind Control has a wonderful little trick for those moments when you catch yourself saying something like, "Looks like there won't be any men in my life this year." Simply say, "Cancel that thought," and replace it with something positive, such as, "I enjoy the wonderful men I choose to have in my life." You do not want to say, "I have an abundance of men in my life," (unless you want that) for surely you will get what you affirm.

Two years ago, my friend Marla was alone and she hated it. She started repeating the affirmation, "I have more men in my life than I know what to do with." Men started coming out of the woodwork! Everywhere she went, she attracted them. She had no time to enjoy the benefits of a relationship with any of them because she "didn't know what to do with them!" Finally, in despair, she threw up her hands and said, "Stop!" Her new affirmation was, "The men in my life are only those I want to spend time with." She now has a few wonderful male friends and is beginning to date one seriously.

In the beginning, not everyone can manifest the way Marla did. Affirmations take time; they don't always happen overnight. Affirmations need to be said over and over until they replace the old negative thought patterns with new positive thoughts. As you practice, you will begin to notice a difference in your life.

A visualization is a mental picture or image that you use in conjunction with a positive affirmation. By using visualizations to create a picture in your mind of what you want, you enhance the power of the affirmation and make it happen more quickly.

Because affirmations and visualizations are thoughts and pictures of what you want to create in your life, your mind may argue at first. It is not important to fully believe the affirmation when you begin, just continue to repeat it. You also do not have to fully believe the visualization, you just have to see it.

Remember, just as your thoughts have created your reality—where you live, the job you have, your bank balance—your thoughts have created your body. You can use affirmations and visualizations to change that creation.

Utilizing Numerous Senses for Reprogramming

Educators know that the more senses you employ in the learning process, the better your chances of retaining what you learn. By combining affirmations and visualizations with movement you are literally reprogramming the muscle tissue memory. Your body holds memory just as your brain does. Saying affirmations while you exercise programs the body to "think" the affirmations whenever you repeat those movements. Your body holds the thought; it is part of you.

I use affirmations in my work with people all the time. Most men and women come to me to get in shape and feel better about themselves. They believe there is something wrong with their bodies, or that they are just keeping bulges at bay by exercising two to three times a week and, often, dieting strenuously. I don't ask them to tell themselves that they are the most beautiful, shapely women or the strongest, most handsome men in the world. I do not encourage them to believe that they have the best bodies in town. That would only set them up for disappointment. I ask them to tell themselves that their bodies are getting better and better every day. I ask them to affirm that beauty and strength are forming and appearing with every movement.

EXERCISE: *How to Affirm a Better Body*

Look at yourself in the mirror and say, "My body is getting better and better every day." What is your response? In the beginning, although you will affirm, "My body is getting better and better every day," you may not believe it, you may not see it. You are accustomed to looking for your faults. You must retrain your eyes—actually you are retraining your mind. On a clean sheet of paper write the affirmation of your choice, then write your subconscious response below it. Repeat the process to fill the entire page.

Example:
Affirmation
My body is getting better and better.

Response
Sure, except for the cellulite on your hips and thighs.

Affirmation
My body is getting better and better.

Response
Don't forget that awful lump just below your buttocks.

Affirmation
My body is getting better and better.

Response
Wait a minute. Your stomach needs to be flatter.

Affirmation
My body is getting better and better.

Response
Well, my waist does look a little tighter.

Affirmation
My body is getting better and better.

Response
I can live with it, it's not so bad.

Affirmation
My body is getting better and better.

Response
I did look good yesterday in that new outfit.

Affirmation
My body is getting better and better.

Response
I am beginning to look better.

Affirmation
My body is getting better and better.

Response
This stuff actually works. I do see a difference. My hips are smaller.

Affirmation
My body is getting better and better.

Response
My body is getting better and better.

Affirmation
My body is getting better and better.

Response
I'm beginning to like my body. It is getting better and better.

As you state and restate the positives, over and over again, watch what happens with both your body and mind. Your body will begin to respond to the positive information your mind is giving it and your mind will begin to enjoy the process of thinking positively. You will feel better and begin to enjoy yourself more.

Sample affirmations:

My body is getting better and better.

Beauty is now forming in every cell in my body.

Every week my waist gets trimmer and trimmer.

I am now beginning to lose the cellulite on the outside of my thighs.

My body is responding to exercise by becoming stronger and more flexible every day.

I am beginning to enjoy my body.

I enjoy my body.

My _____ *is/are perfect.*

I love my _____*!*

My _____ *gives me pleasure to look at.*

Do you notice that these affirmations are not outrageous or impossible? They simply affirm the direction you want to take and aim your mind, as well as your body, in that direction.

Now it is your turn to do the exercise. Do it as many times as you wish, but each time, use only one affirmation for each page of paper. Remember, on a clean sheet of paper, make two columns: *Affirmations* on the left, *Responses* on the right. Proceed with the exercise.

Next, practice the use of visualizations. This will be a more personalized experience because a visualization is your own picture in your mind of how you want your life or your body to be.

Here are two sample visualizations:

Visualization for Your Life

Close your eyes. See a thin veil in front of you. Step through the veil and see yourself taking a path toward your future. Know that the path you take, no matter what it looks like, is the right path. See yourself on the path, moving forward, smiling, feeling free of any fear or concern, knowing you are safe and going in the right direction.

Visualization for Your Body

Close your eyes. Place a mirror before you in your mind's eye. In that mirror see yourself as you would like to be. See yourself with the body, the face, the clothes, the posture, and everything else you would like to have. As you see yourself in that mirror, know that all the cells in your body are responding to your image. As you look at yourself in the mirror, you are becoming exactly what you see. It is YOU you are looking at. Now, step into the mirror. Take the hand of the image you created and begin to merge with your creation. Become one with the image in the mirror and know that it is you.

Using Affirmations and Visualizations in Concert with Exercise

This book is not an exercise book in the conventional sense. What I have discovered is that any exercise or exercise program is good if you do it and if you like it. You decide what works for you.

Affirmations and visualizations can be used in conjunction with any form of exercise. Simply repeat your affirmations as you do what you like to do. Repeat them as you are swimming, or cycling, or to fill in the time when you are walking between the greens at golf. Say affirmations over and over to yourself as you dribble a basketball. Repeat them as you wait for someone to hit a ball to you in the outfield or as you jog down the road.

Some people absolutely hate to exercise. For them, beginning the process of moving at all is the issue that needs to be addressed. If you are very resistant to exercise, begin your affirmations with, "I am willing to begin to move." Movement takes all forms. Walking may be your beginning.

Next, you may want to expand your activities. Decide which body part you want to work on. Check in Chapter Three (The Metaphysics of Body Parts) of this book to see what that part of your body means in your life. Then refer to Chapter Eleven (Affirmations and Visualizations for Body Parts) for affirmations and visualizations relating to that part of your body. Of course, you can make up your own affirmations and visualizations instead of using those we suggest.

EXERCISE: *Defining Your Body Parts*

Example:

> *The body part to work on: my shoulders*
> *What it represents: shoulders carry and support*
> *Affirmation: I release all burdens and carry humor, lightness, and joy. I have perfect shoulders, they are strong and beautiful.*
> *Visualization: I close my eyes and visualize every burden that comes into my life as being encased in a hot air balloon. Each balloon lifts me up rather than weighing me down. I am now freely carried by my former burdens.*

Physical activity for shoulders: swimming, tennis, golf, basket-ball, volleyball, waving my arms in the air, using weights while walking, anything else that moves my shoulders in full rotation.

YOUR TURN

*The body part to work on:*_____

*What it represents:*_____

*Affirmation:*_____

_____

_____

*Visualization:*_____

_____

_____

*Physical activity:*_____

_____

_____

*The body part to work on:*_____

*What it represents:*_____

*Affirmation:*_____

_____

_____

*Visualization:*_____

_____

Physical activity: _____

_____

Use affirmations and visualizations as you swim, ride horseback, play tennis, jog, whatever you like. Don't try to do all the affirmations in this book during a single session. Start with one body part. Choose one that is easy to remember because it strikes a chord with you. Play with it as you exercise and during the day when you are not exercising. Any time you find your mind chatter nagging at you, replace it with your affirmation.

I had one of the more difficult years of my life last year. Nothing seemed to work. There were times when I felt awful, listless, depressed, not wanting to do very much. I couldn't get out of my slump and I was frightened. I had a recurring thought that I would never be happy, successful, or beautiful again. My mind became so negative it was hard to live with it. But I used to go horseback riding; it was the only thing I did that gave me any pleasure. I would ride and be depressed. I had forgotten all about the work I was teaching. I had forgotten about positive thinking and affirmations. I was into my mind chatter and completely under the thumb of my subconscious.

Then one day I simply remembered. I was riding my beautiful horse, Matisse, in Will Rogers State Park. It was a beautiful day, yet I didn't see it. All I could think about was the fact that my career had stopped. I needed to get a television spot or show again, I needed to get publicity, I needed to make the "right" contacts. All this was flying around in my mind, making me feel worse. I remembered all the years in New York when I worked so hard to get what I wanted. All I could think about was the work I had done, the work I was doing, and the work I wanted to do. Then I said, "Wait a minute. Why do you want all these things?" I paused and waited for some revelation, for a golden light to hit me, to show me why I needed to get what I wanted. "You need all these things so that you will have a beautiful house." "I have a beautiful house." "You need all these things so that you can have a horse." "I'm riding my horse." My voice began to get louder, "You need all these things so that you can live the way you want to live." "I **am** living the way I want to live." "YOU NEED ALL THESE THINGS SO THAT YOU CAN WATCH THE SUNSET!!" "IT'S IN FRONT OF YOU, SUZY! YOU ARE WATCHING IT!" At that moment, I knew that I had everything I wanted. I had spent the entire year striving to get something that I already had, but didn't realize it. I had been spending so much time living in the future, that I didn't take time to notice the present.

I realized that in my own life I was not using the tools I was teaching others to use. I started to affirm that my life was beautiful, and that I had everything I wanted. I thought about my body and affirmed that it was toned and flexible. I thought about my finances and affirmed that all my needs were met in present time. I would just ride my horse and affirm, "My life is perfect. I have what I want. My body is beautiful, strong, and toned." I began to visualize myself tanned, toned, and in great shape; smiling and loving life. That's exactly what happened. Pretty soon, my riding time became a time of great joy, a time when I would feel good about myself and my life. And somehow, during this time, my life began to shift. I began to see changes in my life and my body.

I began to notice my thoughts and make them positive. I started to enjoy my work and to acknowledge my enjoyment. The more I affirmed and acknowledged my joy and the condition of my body, the more I enjoyed myself and saw my body change. I received exactly what I affirmed. I still do.

From this day on, consciously choose positive affirmations to become part of your life. Begin by repeating them during exercise periods. Soon you will find yourself using them all the time.

Affirmation

*I use all tools available to me
to change my body and my life.*

11

AFFIRMATIONS AND
VISUALIZATIONS FOR BODY PARTS

"Thought is creative; What you believe to be true becomes manifest in your reality."
— *Werner Erhardt*

*T*he following affirmations and visualizations relate to specific body parts. You may want to refer back to Chapter Three (The Metaphysics of Body Parts) to see what a particular body part means in relation to your life. These affirmations and visualizations are only suggestions; you may want to make up your own. Also, something that is suggested for one body part may make sense to you so strongly that you want to use it for all body parts. If it jumps off the page at you, or you cannot get it out of your head, or it simply feels like the right thing to say, follow your instincts. Repeating endless affirmations that mean nothing to you is an exercise in futility.

Learning to use affirmations and visualizations takes time. For awhile you may have to remind yourself, but if you practice regularly, one day you will find that you automatically repeat affirmations when you need them. They will become part of your life.

I have provided two distinct sets of affirmations and visualizations for each body part. The first affirmation and visualization is designed to heal and change the body part: to bring you a positive relationship with your body, especially the areas where you experience discomfort. These affirmations and visualizations will make you feel good when you look at yourself in the mirror. And you will see positive change in your body without the misery and discomfort you may have experienced in the past.

The second set of affirmations and visualizations relate to the spiritual and symbolic representation of the body part in the world. They can be used to heal body parts or to heal aspects of your life represented by these parts; they are not simply to heal your relationship with the body part. Again, follow your instincts about what seems right for you. Reword affirmations and visualizations to suit your special needs or beliefs.

Always use these in conjunction with your exercise program or favorite physical activity. Eventually you will use affirmations and visualizations in every aspect of your life.

Affirmations and Visualizations for Body Parts

FACE

Affirmation: I have a beautiful face. I love my face. My beauty increases every time I look at my face.

Visualization: Close your eyes. Visualize your face the way you would like it to be. Now visualize your face the way you see it today next to the face you would like to have. See the similarities. See the differences. See your face move toward the face you would love to have, see it meld with that face and see them become one.

Affirmation: I express who I am. It is safe to be me. I love who I am.

Visualization: See yourself smiling, happy with who you are and your way of being in the world. See your face reflect confidence as you greet others in all situations.

EYES

Affirmation: I have beautiful eyes and my vision is perfect. I see everything that I need to see. I love my eyes.

Visualization: Close your eyes. See your eyes in front of you filled with light and love. See your eyes the way you have always wanted them to look. Now overlap the vision of your eyes with the beautiful eyes the way that you have always wanted them to look. Let your eyes and the image become one.

Affirmation: I see myself, my eyes, and my body with love and joy. I see the perfection of my life. I see the perfection of the world around me.

Visualization: See yourself with a bow and arrow aiming at a row of targets in the distance. Each target represents a life issue. Your eyes are able to see them clearly and honestly. See yourself shooting at each target and getting a bull's-eye every time, knowing that the life issues that the targets represent are healing quickly and perfectly.

NOSE

Affirmation: My nose is perfect. I love my nose.

Visualization: Close your eyes. See your nose the way you have always wanted it to be. See your nose the way you think it is today. See the two pictures blending, becoming one. See your nose becoming the way you have always wanted it to be.

Affirmation: I love and approve of myself. I recognize my own true worth and my intuitive ability. I am wonderful.

Visualization: See yourself standing before a crowd. All of the people look like you and they are all beautiful. See the crowd of beautiful people recognizing you as the best looking of them all. Step forward and be seen for the beautiful, handsome being you are.

MOUTH

Affirmation: My mouth is beautiful. It is perfect for me and who I am.

Visualization: Close your eyes. See yourself in a mirror. Look closely at your mouth. See your mouth as perfect as all the other parts of your face. Smile in recognition of your beauty.

Affirmation: I nourish myself with love.

Visualization: See and hear yourself in conversation with a good friend. You say all the right things at the right time. Know that your mouth is perfect and always speaks appropriately.

CHEEKS

Affirmation: I have beautiful cheeks. They are wonderful to look at and to touch.

Visualization: Close your eyes. See yourself in a mirror. Look at your face. See the lines of your cheeks exactly as you want them to be. See yourself smiling and knowing that your cheeks reflect the perfect you.

Affirmation: I am good enough. I accept myself exactly as I am. I love myself.

Visualization: See yourself in front of a large audience of your peers. Your cheeks are blushing happily as you graciously accept an award for being perfect exactly as you are.

CHIN

Affirmation: I have a strong, beautiful chin. I love my chin.
Visualization: Close your eyes. See yourself in a mirror, look at your chin. Turn your face from side to side to examine the beauty of the lines of your chin. See your chin as perfect and know that this is who you are.

Affirmation: It is safe to be who I am. I celebrate my power and my vulnerability.
Visualization: See yourself walking down the street. As others pass by you, notice that they admire how your chin is held high and reflects the strength and confidence you have in yourself.

EARS

Affirmation: My ears are perfect. I have beautiful ears.
Visualization: Close your eyes. See yourself in a mirror, look at your ears. See your ears exactly as you would like them to be. See your ears as they are. Now see them melding, becoming one; your ears are becoming exactly as you would like them to be. See your ears as perfect.

Affirmation: Harmony surrounds me. I listen with love to the pleasant and the good. I am a center for love. I hear with love.
Visualization: See yourself listening to your favorite performer at a live concert. Bless the ability of your ears to bring you such enrichment of life and always know that what you hear will be heard at the right time and be perfect for you.

HAIR

Affirmation: I have beautiful hair. It is the perfect color, thickness, and style.
Visualization: Close your eyes. See yourself fixing your hair in the morning. See how easily it falls into place with minimum fuss. Admire your hair and know that it is just right for you.

Affirmation: I am perfect just the way I am. I trust myself. I trust life.
Visualization: See yourself smiling into the mirror. You are running your fingers through your hair and admiring its texture. You know that it reflects your masculinity/femininity perfectly for you.

NECK AND SHOULDERS

NECK

Affirmation: My neck is strong and beautiful. It moves easily without tension.

Visualization: Close your eyes. See a swan gliding across a quiet pond. Notice how graceful, flexible, and perfect a neck it has. See your neck as graceful, flexible, and perfect for you just as the swan's is for it.

Affirmation: I easily see all sides of issues and see endless ways of doing things. I am safe and peaceful in my life.
Visualization: See a giraffe eating leaves from a tree. Notice how easily his neck supports his head and how fluidly it moves. See your neck move just as easily and freely without pain. Know that, like your neck, you are able to face all issues from all sides and accomplish what is perfect for you.

SHOULDERS

Affirmation: My shoulders are strong and beautiful. They are upright and tension-free.
Visualization: Close your eyes. See yourself with the shoulders you want. See yourself smiling, laughing, happy with your posture, strength, and beauty.

Affirmation: My burdens are light; they support my growth. I choose to allow all my experiences to be joyous and loving.
Visualization: See yourself walking down the street. Your shoulders are strong and easily able to carry your burdens. Each burden is like a helium balloon. One by one they are being lifted and carried off by the wind. You no longer have to carry them as burdens, but can walk with them as opportunities.

ARMS

UPPER ARMS

Affirmation: My upper arms are beautiful, strong, toned, and firm.
Visualization: Close your eyes. See your upper arms as they are. Now see your upper arms becoming the upper arms you would like them to be. Visualize the lines, the tone, and the firmness.

Affirmation: I lovingly hold and embrace my experiences with ease and joy.
Visualization: See yourself in a beautiful, peaceful mountain setting. You stretch your arms joyfully and easily over your head as if to greet the world. You know your arms are strong and are able to lovingly embrace all issues that come up in your life.

ELBOWS

Affirmation: My elbows are perfect. They bend and straighten with ease.
Visualization: Close your eyes. See yourself with beautiful elbows. See them bend and straighten with ease. There is no pain or discomfort. See yourself smiling, knowing you have perfect elbows.

Affirmation: I easily flow with new experiences, new directions, and new changes.

Visualization: See yourself participating in a variety of sports that utilize the elbows (archery, bowling, horseshoes, etc.). As you change sports, your elbows are able to adapt effortlessly and painlessly. Know that, like your elbows, you can handle all changes that occur in your life with great ease.

LOWER ARMS

Affirmation: My lower arms are beautiful and strong.

Visualization: Close your eyes. See your lower arms exactly the way you want them to be. They are toned, strong, and beautiful.

Affirmation: I celebrate the experiences in my life. I hold them with joy and ease.

Visualization: See yourself juggling four balls in front of a small audience at the beach. Each ball represents a life issue for you. You instruct someone to toss you another ball. They do and you continue juggling with ease. Another ball is tossed to you and you now effortlessly juggle all six balls. The crowd applauds and you know that your life will always be in perfect balance and never overwhelm you.

WRISTS

Affirmation: I have beautiful, strong, and flexible wrists.

Visualization: Close your eyes. See your beautiful wrists, able to move with ease. See them strong, toned, and flexible.

Affirmation: I handle all my experiences with wisdom, with love, and with ease.

Visualization: See yourself playing a rapid game of ping-pong. Your wrists move fluidly and easily. You know that you will handle life as fluidly and easily as your wrists move.

HANDS AND FINGERS

HANDS

Affirmation: I have beautiful, strong, flexible hands.

Visualization: Close your eyes. See your hands as you would like them to be. See them becoming stronger, more flexible, and beautiful.

Affirmation: I handle all my experiences with love and joy. I hold my life with ease.

Visualization: See yourself as the host of a fabulous party. As your guests arrive you greet each of them with a firm handshake. Your guests notice how confident you are and how easily and skillfully you are able to manage your life.

FINGERS

Thumb

Affirmation: My thumb is perfect.

Visualization: Close your eyes. In your mind, look at your thumb. See it perfect, strong, flexible, and able to move and straighten with ease.

Affirmation: My mind is at peace. I am doing exactly what I want to do in my life.

Visualization: See yourself hitchhiking by the side of a country road on a crisp, clear morning. You are joyfully heading towards a new avenue, a new realm of satisfaction. You know that you will go exactly where you want easily and effortlessly.

Index Finger

Affirmation: My index finger is strong, beautiful, and flexible.

Visualization: Close your eyes. See your index finger able to move and straighten with ease. It is strong and flexible.

Affirmation: I am willing and able to handle all of my life. I follow my intuition and my ambition with ease.

Visualization: See yourself shooting at targets in a carnival shooting gallery. Each target you hit represents a personal ambition that you have. As your index finger pulls the trigger on the gun you know that you will achieve your goals with as little effort as it takes to knock down the target.

Middle Finger

Affirmation: My middle finger is beautiful, strong, and flexible.

Visualization: Close your eyes. See your middle finger able to move and straighten with ease. It is strong and flexible.

Affirmation: I have integrity in my life. I love my choices and know that I am right.

Visualization: You are a speaker at a victory rally for a cause you feel strongly about. You have just given a rousing speech. As you give the "victory" sign, the crowd cheers loudly and you know that your sense of right and wrong will always be in perfect balance as you go through life.

Ring Finger

Affirmation: My ring finger is beautiful, strong, and flexible.

Visualization: Close your eyes. See your ring finger able to move and straighten with ease. It is strong and flexible.

Affirmation: I am peacefully loving. I am creative. I express with love who I am. I relate to others with ease and understanding.

Visualization: See yourself in a workshop creating a ring for your finger. The ideas flow to you swiftly, each one more creative than the last, until you create the perfect design. You know that your creative powers and self-expression are in peak form and will always be there when you need them.

Little Finger

Affirmation: My little finger is beautiful, strong, and flexible.

Visualization: Close your eyes. See your little finger able to move and straighten with ease. It is strong and flexible.

Affirmation: I am myself with the family of life. My relationships are loving. I communicate with ease and joy.

Visualization: See yourself as a magician performing great feats of magic with every wave of your hand. Your creativity is limitless as you keep your audience spellbound with every trick you do. You know that your creativity and self-expression will always be in abundant supply for you whenever you need them.

THE BACK

Upper Back

Affirmation: My upper back is strong and beautiful. I carry joy and move with ease.

Visualization: Close your eyes. See yourself with the upper back you have always wanted. See your upper back becoming the way you have envisioned it. Know that you have the perfect upper back.

Affirmation: I love and approve of myself. Life supports and loves me. I am safe loving and safe being loved.

Visualization: See yourself transporting some heavy boxes up a stairway. Since the boxes have a carrying strap on them, the easiest way to carry them is on your upper back. As you take each box up the stairs you know that your upper back will always get you through your life safely and supportively.

Mid-Back

Affirmation: My middle back is strong, toned, flexible, and beautiful. It is smooth and exactly the way I want it to be.

Visualization: Close your eyes. See your middle back strong, toned, flexible, and smooth. See the firm and gentle lines of the muscles. See your middle back exactly as you want it to be.

Affirmation: I release the past. I am free to move forward with love in my heart. I am safe in the freedom of my life.

Visualization: See yourself in your living area getting ready to do the most graceful backbend you have ever done. As your hands reach over your head toward the floor you have absolutely no fears that your back will get stuck before you reach the floor. Like your middle back, you know that life issues will never keep you hemmed in with feelings of guilt or fear.

Lower Back

Affirmation: My lower back is perfect, strong, and flexible. My lower back moves and holds me in comfort and ease.
Visualization: Close your eyes. See yourself standing and then moving with ease and comfort, knowing your lower back is perfect, pain-free, and in good condition.

Affirmation: I trust life and am supported by life. I always have everything I need. I am safe.
Visualization: See yourself horseback riding on a beautiful country estate. As you gallop across a windswept meadow, you notice how strongly and steadily your lower back supports you with each gallop of your horse. You joyfully acknowledge that you will never have any fears of support in your lifetime.

CHEST AND BREASTS

The Chest

Affirmation: My chest is beautiful, well-defined, strong, and powerful.
Visualization: Close your eyes. See yourself with your perfect chest. Your shoulders are straight and the lines of your chest are toned, smooth, and strong.

Affirmation: I love my life. I am safe. I love being loved. I love giving and receiving. I take in and utilize all of life's loving experiences.
Visualization: See yourself on a wonderful hiking trip with several of your best friends. High on a mountaintop, you stop for a moment to breathe in the fresh air. As you take several deep breaths you can feel the life force from the earth and the love force from your friends go through your chest and into the very center of your being.

The Breasts

Affirmation: My breasts are beautiful. They are perfect just the way they are.
Visualization: Close your eyes. See your breasts as you would like them to be. See yourself having the breasts you want. See yourself smiling, happy with your breasts.

Affirmation: I am balanced in giving and receiving love. I lovingly allow myself to be nurtured. I love to receive as much as I give.
Visualization: See yourself standing in front of a mirror getting ready for a fancy dinner party. The outfit you have chosen shows off your breasts to their best advantage. You are comfortable with this level of sensuality and femininity. You know that your breasts are beautiful. It is comfortable for you to see your beauty and for you to nurture yourself and others.

MIDRIFF AND WAIST

Midriff

Affirmation: My midriff is perfect, strong, toned, smooth, and flexible.
Visualization: Close your eyes. See yourself with the torso that you want. See the lines of your midriff. Feel your midriff's strength and flexibility. See yourself toned and happy.

Affirmation: I am safe to feel all of my emotions. My emotions love me and allow me to experience life more fully with love and joy.
Visualization: See yourself at a small informal party with a close group of friends. You are playing a harmless version of "Truth or Dare." When your turn comes up, you discover that you have to do a belly dance. As you do your dance, any negative emotion that had come up out of embarrassment now turns to pride as your friends comment how flat, toned, and attractive your midriff is. You know that you will always be able to deal with your emotions easily and effortlessly.

Waist

Affirmation: My waist is perfect, smooth, toned, strong, and flexible.
Visualization: Close your eyes. See yourself with your perfect waist, bending and turning with ease. See the smooth lines. Feel your waist's strength and flexibility. See yourself smiling, happy with your waist.

Affirmation: I move with ease in my life, able to turn in any direction with joy and comfort.
Visualization: See yourself in a dance contest at a "60s Party." You decide to do the "twist," and as you compete in the final round, your waist is so flexible, strong, and able to turn that you win the competition easily. You know that, like your waist, you will always have the ability to be flexible and to see the different angles of life.

STOMACH (ABDOMEN)

Affirmation: My stomach is beautiful, strong, and toned. It is perfect and I love it.
Visualization: Close your eyes. See yourself with the stomach you have always wanted. Now see the stomach you have becoming the stomach you have always wanted to have. See yourself loving your stomach, happy with it, pleased with the way it looks and feels.

Affirmation: I am safe to fully digest all that comes to me in my life. I am safe in every situation and with every new idea. It is okay for me to follow my inner knowing. I love my creativity. I love my sexuality.

Visualization: See yourself as a small child hanging upside-down from monkey bars at a playground. You can creatively move around and you intuitively know that no harm will come to you. Your stomach muscles function perfectly and pull you up when you want them to. See yourself change into the adult you are now. Your stomach is even stronger, tighter, and more beautiful than it was when you were a child and you are more creative and have a greater sense of inner knowing now than you ever did before.

HIPS AND BUTTOCKS

Hips

Affirmation: My hips are perfect, strong, toned, shapely, and flexible.
Visualization: Close your eyes. See yourself with hips exactly the way you want them. See the hips you have becoming the hips you want. See yourself loving your hips.

Affirmation: I am free to move forward, in perfect balance, with joy and laughter. There is joy in every day and in everything I do.
Visualization: See yourself in Hawaii doing a Hula show. You are the star performer and as you dance, your hips move easily and in perfect balance with each other. The crowd applauds as you display the exotic hip techniques that you have become famous for. You know that, like your hips, your life will always be balanced in movement and creativity.

Buttocks

Affirmation: I love my buttocks, they are firm, toned, strong, and beautiful.
Visualization: Close your eyes. See yourself with the perfect rear end. See it exactly as you want it to be. Feel yourself having that perfect rear end. Love your buttocks for becoming exactly what you want them to be.

Affirmation: I am safe in my power. I hold my power and use it wisely, and with love. I am safe in my power and with the power of others.
Visualization: See yourself in a country setting. You are exercising by running up a hill. You feel powerful as your buttocks work together with your legs to take you up the hill easily and in perfect stride. Running down the hill you know that you will never have a fear of your own or anyone else's power.

LEGS

Thighs

Affirmation: My thighs are beautiful, strong, toned, and flexible. They move with grace and ease.

Visualization: Close your eyes. See yourself with thighs exactly as you want them. See your own thighs becoming the thighs you have created. You are happy to have such attractive thighs.

Affirmation: I forgive all childhood trespasses, real and imagined, and go forth to positive feelings. I love life and enjoy my experiences, past and present.

Visualization: See yourself skiing down a mountain slope on a crisp, clear day. As you move forward, your thighs bend easily with each turn. You know that the strength in your thighs represents your inner strength and your ability to move forward.

Knees

Affirmation: I love my knees. They are beautiful, strong, shapely, and flexible.

Visualization: Close your eyes. See yourself with perfect knees, exactly the way you want them to be. Feel your knees be what you want. Love your knees.

Affirmation: My life is balanced. I work and I play equally, with joy and delight. I bend and flow with ease.

Visualization: See yourself on a surfboard in the dark blue waters of Hawaii. A huge wave has come up and you are riding it back to the shore. Your knees are strong and flexible. They always keep you in perfect balance with the wave. You know that your life will always be balanced and flexible.

Calves

Affirmation: I love my calves, they are beautiful, strong, toned, and flexible.

Visualization: Close your eyes. See yourself with calves exactly as you want them to be. See your calves becoming the calves you want to have. Feel your body changing. Love your calves.

Affirmation: I move forward in my life safely and with ease. I am safe now and in the future.

Visualization: See yourself as a tightrope walker, high above an audience at a circus. As you successfully move forward across the rope, your lower legs are firm and solid. They take you across the rope perfectly. You know that you will always have the ability to move forward in life without fear or trepidation.

Ankles

Affirmation: I have beautiful ankles. They are strong, toned and flexible.

Visualization: Close your eyes. See yourself with beautiful ankles, strong, toned, and flexible. See your present ankles becoming the ankles you see in your mind. Know that you have beautiful ankles.

Affirmation: I am safe. I move with ease and flexibility and communicate freely. All is well with me in the world.

Visualization: See yourself as a ballet dancer in a famous ballet company. As you stride across the stage, your ankles bend and flex with perfect grace. They take you through leaps and pirouettes without any discomfort or pain. You beam as the audience applauds and you know that you will always have the gift to receive, as well as give, pleasure.

FEET AND TOES

Feet

Affirmation: I love my feet. They are beautiful, strong, and flexible.
Visualization: Close your eyes. See yourself with perfect feet; feet that are strong, flexible, and able to carry you with ease and comfort.

Affirmation: I love my life and the way I choose to live. I am safe following my dreams. I love taking care of myself. All is well and perfect in my life.

Visualization: See yourself dancing like Fred Astaire or Ginger Rogers on a beautiful stage. Your feet move freely and marvelously in time with the music. The way you move makes you feel elegant and beautiful. Your confidence soars! You know that you can always follow your dreams without fear of failure and that you will never be so busy that you cannot take time for yourself.

Toes

Big Toe
Affirmation: My big toe is perfect. I love my big toe.
Visualization: Close your eyes. See your big toe, the perfect shape and size, feeling good and able to move with ease.

Affirmation: I handle all details of what I want to do with ease and joy. I follow through with everything easily. It is simple for me to leave nothing unnoticed or unfulfilled.

Visualization: See yourself in a ballet class. You stand on your toes in an "en pointe" exercise and your big toe is strong and supportive even when you put the rest of your weight on it. As you come down off your toes, you check to make sure your big toe is not hurt. You know that you will always pay attention to details in your life so that nothing remains unfulfilled.

Second Toe
Affirmation: My second toe is perfect. I love my second toe.
Visualization: Close your eyes. See your second toe. It is the perfect shape and size, feeling good, and able to move with ease.

Affirmation: I am skilled at handling my life and follow my intuition with ease and commitment. My projects are easy to handle, money now makes sense and is easy to have and to work with.
Visualization: See yourself leading a scout troop for an overnight stay in the woods. Your feet are strong and sure of themselves as they lead the way to the perfect spot for your camp. The children feel very safe with your leadership abilities and later that night around the campfire, they toast you with hot chocolate as the best leader of all.

Middle Toe
Affirmation: My middle toe is perfect. I love my middle toe.
Visualization: Close your eyes. See your middle toe. It is the perfect shape and size. It feels good, and is able to move with ease.

Affirmation: I live in integrity, loving truth, and honoring my way of being in the world. I am perfect just the way I am.
Visualization: See yourself walking down a crowded city sidewalk. Suddenly, a purse snatcher grabs an older woman's purse next to you and runs away with it. You immediately start running after the thief without concern for your personal safety. You know that you will be safe. You catch up with the thief and take the purse back. The thief runs away empty-handed. You return the purse to its rightful owner. You thank your feet for being so quick and powerful; you thank yourself for knowing the difference between right and wrong.

Fourth Toe
Affirmation: My fourth toe is perfect. I love my fourth toe.
Visualization: Close your eyes. See your fourth toe. It is the perfect shape and size. It feels good, and is able to move with ease.

Affirmation: I express myself creatively, with joy and clarity. I am safe and strong, able to maintain my autonomy while I am in relationship with others.
Visualization: See yourself as an artist with the most outstanding abilities. Anything you choose to do you do with great style and expression, even fingerpainting with your toes! See a finished product of your artistic abilities. It utilizes your favorite colors. It is just the right size. It communicates your thoughts and feelings perfectly. You know that you will always have creative powers that are perfectly suited for you.

Little Toe
Affirmation: My little toe is perfect. I love my little toe.
Visualization: Close your eyes. See your little toe. It is the perfect shape and size. It feels good, and is able to move with ease.

Affirmation: I love to communicate and do so with joy and ease. My relationships are perfect. I am safe loving and being loved.

Visualization: See yourself in a wonderful natural setting walking with someone (maybe a family member or personal friend) you have had difficulty communicating with in the past. As you walk, notice how easily and honestly you talk with each other. You both feel a great barrier is broken through as you talk about the difficult times that your relationship has survived. You resolve your differences and give your relationship a new, deeper purpose. You know that you will always be able to communicate your feelings and thoughts clearly to anyone you meet.

OTHERS

Cellulite

Affirmation: I love my body. I love the texture of my skin, the lines of my limbs, and the toned quality of every part of me.

Visualization: Close your eyes. See yourself perfect, exactly the way you want to be. See your body releasing all the stored "fat" in the cellulite. See the fat become smooth and toned. You are happy with yourself and the way you look.

Affirmation: I live life joyously, happy with myself, and with my experiences. I allow myself the joys and pleasures of life with delight. I am right in what I choose for myself. Life is a blessing and a joy.

Visualization: See yourself in your last unresolved angry situation. You are unable to vent your true feelings and you feel them bottling up inside of you. With these bottled-up feelings you run to the top of a lovely, green, solitary hill. Running has made you feel good and has already dissipated some of the anger. You let go with a loud, piercing yell, which releases the rest of it. You feel wonderful and you look wonderful. You know that you can work off your cellulite as easily as you can work off your anger.

Bones

Affirmation: My bones are strong. They carry me with strength and ease. I have perfect posture and look beautiful.

Visualization: Close your eyes. See yourself as strong, toned, and beautiful, standing straight, with perfect posture, feeling good, and loving yourself.

Affirmation: My life is perfect. I love my life and the way I live it.

Visualization: See yourself having a complete body x-ray. It is perfectly safe and you are able to see all of your bones at once. You marvel at their intricacy and function. They have brought the perfect structure into your body and you know that your life will always be as perfectly structured wherever you are.

Fat

Affirmation: I love my fat. It protects me and keeps me safe. It has done a great job and now it can go on vacation permanently.

Visualization: Close your eyes. See yourself releasing your fat. See the lines of your body slowly moving, shaping your body exactly how you want it to look. Love your body in every stage of its being. See yourself safe and beautiful in every way.

Affirmation: I am safe in every aspect and feeling in my life. I easily express and release my emotions with joy and in safety.

Visualization: See yourself in your last fearful situation. Know that fear is a valid feeling, but like most feelings, it must be resolved. See yourself resolving this fear in the way you think best. Know that you are safe, and as you calmly let go of the fear, let go of the fat that has served to protect you. See the fat leave your body. See yourself courageous and confident.

Skin

Affirmation: I have perfect skin. It is beautiful, smooth, and toned. I love my skin.

Visualization: Close your eyes. See yourself exactly as you would like to be. See yourself smiling, radiating beauty and joy.

Affirmation: I am safe being me. I love myself and who I am. I enjoy the richness of life, I experience with delight my senses; hearing, seeing, feeling, tasting, and smelling. I trust my senses and know I am right.

Visualization: See yourself standing unclothed in a wonderful box of blue light. The blue light warms and caresses the entire skin of your body. As it caresses, it also repairs and smooths. It brings out the best colors in your skin and you know that the skin marks the individual that is you. You are unique and you joyfully accept your individuality.

Muscles

Affirmation: I have strong, flexible, well-conditioned, well-toned muscles. They move with ease, strength, and fluidity. I love my beautiful muscles.

Visualization: Close your eyes. See yourself, strong and graceful, moving through your life with joy and ease. See yourself physically able to do anything that you want.

Affirmation: I love my life and my freedom to move in any direction with ease and safety.

Visualization: Imagine your own skeleton lying helpless on your bed. Now slip some muscles on these bones, just as you would put on a new outfit. See how perfectly your muscles fit your bones. They hold your bones together and give them the structure that they need to move freely and painlessly. You feel safe knowing that your life will always have the perfect structure within its framework.

SPECIFIC PROBLEMS

Flexibility

Affirmation: I am flexible. I move with grace and fluidity. I love the way I move.

Visualization: Close your eyes. See yourself like a dancer, able to move with grace and fluidity. See yourself flexible, well-toned, and happy with your body.

Affirmation: I love my life and all that it offers me. I enjoy new directions. Life is a joyous kaleidoscope of change.

Visualization: See yourself in a local decathlon. As you go through each event, you marvel at how adaptable your body is in anything you do. Your flexibility knows no bounds. You are triumphant in every event and you know that your body reflects your own ability to be flexible in any given situation.

Pain

Affirmation: My body feels great. I love my body, it loves me.

Visualization: Close your eyes. See yourself happy. See your body feeling great, able to do everything. See yourself enjoying your life and the things you do every day. See your body looking healthy.

Affirmation: I forgive myself for everything I think I have done, real or imagined, that I feel guilty about. I love myself and my way of being in the world.

Visualization: See yourself in a personal guilt-inducing situation. Know that the past is done with and that you are only living in the present. You have no need for any more guilt or pain for something you cannot change. It is over. You know that guilt is a valid emotion, but must now be replaced by a more positive one like self-forgiveness and self-love. You know that guilt and pain will never have a permanent home in your body.

Stiffness

Affirmation: My body moves with grace and ease. My muscles are flexible, well-toned, and in good condition.

Visualization: Close your eyes. See yourself moving with ease. See all your limbs moving gracefully. See your back and shoulders relaxed either while still or in motion. See yourself happy with your ability to move easily.

Affirmation: I love new ideas. I am always open to new ideas and beliefs to enhance my life.

Visualization: See yourself made out of wax. You are cold and lying in the sun to warm up. At first you are completely stiff, but as the sun permeates your body, you begin to loosen up and become more flexible. Your stiffness continues to disappear until you can move in any direction you choose. You know that you will always be open to new ideas or beliefs.

Spasm

Affirmation: My body feels good, relaxed, and in good condition. My muscles move with ease. They are fluid, strong, and relaxed.

Visualization: Close your eyes. See yourself smiling and comfortable. See your muscles relaxed, able to do what they need to do comfortably and easily.

Affirmation: I am safe. It is a joy to be alive. I am okay just the way I am.

Visualization: See yourself as a spinning top, going faster as you tighten with fear. Now see these fears coming unglued and being flung away by your spinning motion. As each fear is tossed away, you begin to slow down. The tightness is disappearing, and with it, the need for the spasms. Your body feels loose and free and can never be shocked by tightness or spasms again. Whenever you feel the tightness coming up, you see yourself spinning and throwing your fears aside. This always slows you down and gives you the comfort that you need to function with ease.

Affirmation

*I lovingly affirm and visualize the
strength and beauty within me.
I choose to be the perfect me.*

12

LOVE YOUR GOOD LOOKS, ACKNOWLEDGE YOURSELF, BECOME WHAT YOU WANT TO BE

"A thing of beauty is a joy forever;
Its loveliness increases; it will never
Pass into nothingness."
— *John Keats*

*B*eginning today, every day and forever more, at least three times a day, look at yourself in the mirror and tell yourself how good you look. It does not matter what your mind says, keep saying how good you look. Find things about yourself that you really like. Focus on them. Tell yourself you look fabulous. Very quickly, your mind chatter will get quieter and your belief in your own good looks will improve.

I had a wonderful experience several years ago, when I started doing this. One bright, spring day, as I was walking down a New York City street window-shopping, I saw a beautiful woman reflected in the glass. When I stopped to look at the woman, I realized it was me! Also, around that time, I noticed that other people started telling me I was beautiful. People would ask me if I had been on vacation or if I was in love. Sometimes they would ask if I had changed my hair, or lost weight. All this time I had not gained or lost a pound, changed my hair style or my makeup, or met a man, and I was working harder than ever. I had not even bought new clothes. Basically, I was the same person, only my beliefs about myself had changed.

I have to confess there are times when I forget to be positive with myself or I begin to allow my critical voice to become louder than my affirmative voice. But, as long as I believe in myself and in my own beauty, the results show in a positive way in my life and my body.

When I lecture, I always ask my audiences, "How many of you look in the mirror and tell yourself how good you look?" There are always a few who do, but mostly I watch people look nervously at each other, and I hear laughter, "What, are you kidding?"

In one of my workshops, we were doing the following exercise: Look at yourself in a mirror. Start with your face. Find something nice about your face. I watched a woman named Eleanor as she avoided looking at her face in the mirror for forty-five minutes. When I approached her, she said, "I can't do it. Whenever I look at my face all I see are my cheeks, which I hate. I've never been able to look at my face. Even when I put my makeup on, I avoid looking at my face. I can't see anything I like, let alone something beautiful about it." I asked her to shift her vision to her eyes. As she looked, I asked her to examine the color and the shape of her eyes without looking at any other part. She did this, and soon tears began to slowly fall from her eyes. She stammered, "They are beautiful. I've never seen them before." By really seeing her eyes for the first time, Eleanor began the process of healing her relationship with her own face. She began to see her own beauty.

Because so many of us have been trained to see the negative, we must consciously begin to focus on ourselves differently. Stay away from the things you do not like about your body until you can fully acknowledge what you do like.

The following exercise is similar to the one you did in Chapter Four, but instead of looking at how your mind berates you with negative thoughts, you will celebrate your emerging health, good looks, and positive feelings. This exercise may seem difficult or uncomfortable at first, but stick with it.

EXERCISE: *Celebrate Your Good Looks*

Stand in front of a mirror (naked, if you can). Tell yourself how beautiful you are. If you hear mind chatter, stop, listen to it, and turn it around into something positive. Now, find one thing you like about your body. It might be the texture of your skin or the way your shoulders slope. I love my hips. I always start with them. Then I go on from there.

> *Once you find an area or areas you can acknowledge, do so. Tell yourself how beautiful that part of you is. Again, it does not matter what your mind says. Thank it for sharing, turn-around the thought into something positive and keep going.*

You will begin to notice right away that your mind chatter is becoming quieter. But remember, it took years to develop these beliefs about yourself, and it will take awhile to undo them.

EXERCISE: *Mirror Work*

> *You will find it helpful to keep a small hand mirror with you at all times. Right now, take out that mirror, look at yourself and say, "I love you." That's all. Listen to your negative mind chatter; do not argue with it, just listen. Again, look at yourself in the mirror and say, "I really love you."*

Once you develop a relationship with yourself in the mirror, you will find that you can depend on a dialogue between yourself and the mirror to always tell you the truth. You can learn your innermost needs by talking to yourself in the mirror. If something unpleasant happens to you, go to the mirror and talk to yourself. Say, it is really alright. The event will pass, but the relationship you have with yourself will remain forever.

Louise L. Hay told me a story about when she was working on a new book. Somehow she pushed the wrong buttons on her computer and lost three chapters she had just finished. Without hesitation she ran to the mirror and said, "I love you. It's all right. Don't worry, you didn't mean to do it. I forgive you and truly love you." She did not get mad at herself, or blame herself, or hold a secret grudge against herself. In this way, she keeps a wonderful love of herself. And, of course, this allows for everyone else to love her, too.

> *"Mirrors are one of the most powerful tools when we want to make positive changes in our lives. Just looking in the mirror, telling yourself positive things, or doing 'mirror work,' as I call it, cuts down the time involved in changing.*
>
> *I have seen numerous people change their lives by merely looking in the mirror and saying, 'I love you, I really love you.' At first, it seems untrue or even weird. This exercise can bring up anger or sadness or even fear. Still, if we continue to do this simple affirmation every time we are in front of a mirror, our inner energy begins to shift, releasing destructive thoughts and behaviors. In time, we find that we really do love ourselves."*
>
> *— Louise L. Hay*

Start now to use the mirror. You will find that the more you do it, the easier it gets. As you discover more and more things to acknowledge about yourself, more positive things will come into your life, and you will truly begin to like who you are.

I used to think that acknowledgements had to be celebrations of something huge or something tangible. But that kind of thinking overlooks a lot of potential for feeling good by acknowledging all the wonderful "little" things that you do. It also creates a standard that makes it almost impossible for them to be noticed.

I always attempt to acknowledge things that are not obvious, and things I used to take for granted. I was expected to make my bed, so I never acknowledged myself for doing it. If I left the bed unmade I would nag and berate myself for being a slob, but I let an opportunity to praise myself go by each time I made it.

EXERCISE: *Loving Yourself*

This is probably my favorite exercise. Select the part of your body that you like the least and talk about all the good things it does for you. Describe this part of your body in the most glowing terms.

Example:

I find it difficult to love my rear end, but on the positive side: My rear end is loyal, it follows me everywhere. It cushions my seat bones when I sit down. It stores food in case of famine. It fills out my clothes with firm, full lines.

YOUR TURN

*I find it difficult to love my*_____

*but on the positive side:*_____

_____

_____

_____

You can have a good time with this exercise, and shift your energy from anger and disappointment (in yourself) to humor and love (with yourself).

When I began to do this exercise, I soon discovered that the shape of my rear end was changing and I began to like it. Now, it has gotten to be quite lovely and I can do the positive exercise of saying that I love it without a lot of mind chatter.

You will find, after awhile, that your body will become more and more beautiful to you, that those areas which caused you consternation in the past are changing. They are changing in your eyes and on your body. Clothes will fit you differently and people will compliment you in ways they never have before. It may seem strange, but it works.

Remember, you are doing two things here: you are changing your beliefs about yourself and you are working on changing your body. As you learn to love yourself, if you back up that love with a practical program, you will get results. But remember, MetaFitness will only work if you do it: evaluate your body, commit to make a change, set your goals and follow through, then acknowledge your accomplishments and yourself.

Do you notice how often you are on time, or do you only notice when you are late? Do you notice when your desk is neat, or only when it is messy? Do you congratulate yourself for getting work done on time, or yell at yourself when it is late? Do you thank yourself because you stop eating when you are full, or do you wait until you are stuffed, feel uncomfortable, and then get upset with yourself?

EXERCISE: *What I Take For Granted*

Make a list of what you take for granted and what you allow your critical voice to use against you.

Example:
What I take for granted:
1. Being on time.
I hardly notice when I am on time. I am supposed to be on time. It is expected of me. But when I am late my critical voice has a heyday; I yell and scream at myself inside my mind.
2. Cleaning the house.
I take it for granted that my house is always clean. And when it is not, my critical voice nags and nags at me; it points out what a slob I am. My critical voice tells me that other people will think less of me when my home is messy.
3. Taking my keys out of the ignition when I park my car.
This may seem routine, but what happens when you forget? One time I locked my keys in the car, with the motor running, on Broadway and 86th Street in New York City. I was mortified. I yelled at myself all the way home to get my other set. By the time the drama was over, I felt awful. Another time, on my way to the airport I stopped to get a sandwich (I don't like airline food) and locked my keys in the car. I calmly noticed what I had done and called AAA. The whole incident was handled in less than 10 minutes with no drama, and I felt proud of myself instead of angry.
Begin to notice the things you take for granted. You will like yourself more, and enjoy everything you do, rather than just waiting for the big stuff to acknowledge.

More examples of what I take for granted are:
1. *Getting up in the morning.*
2. *Getting stamps on all the bills and getting them in the mail box (with checks inside).*
3. *Not getting up in the morning if you need a rest.*
4. *Working on your thighs even if you cannot see the difference. (Especially if you cannot see the difference.)*
5. *Cleaning your desk.*
6. *Leaving food on your plate when you have had enough to eat.*

What I take for granted:_____

What I allow my critical voice to use against me:_____

_____

What I take for granted:_____

What I allow my critical voice to use against me:_____

_____

What I take for granted:_____

What I allow my critical voice to use against me:_____

_____

What I take for granted:_____

What I allow my critical voice to use against me:_____

_____

EXERCISE: *Acknowledging Yourself*

Every evening this week do the following exercise.
Ten things I want to acknowledge myself for doing today:

Example:
1. *Finished chapters 11 through 14.*
2. *Got my son's Christmas presents.*
3. *Mailed my son's Christmas presents.*
4. *Got a new accountant.*
5. *Sat in front of the fire and did nothing for 15 minutes.*
6. *Ate well.*

    7. Spent time painting.
    8. Got my car washed.
    9. Turned the heat off when I left the house.
    10. Took time to look in the mirror and say "I love you."

YOUR TURN

1. _____

2. _____

3. _____

4. _____

5. _____

6. _____

7. _____

8. _____

9. _____

10. _____

Perform this exercise as close to bedtime as possible so you can end the day with positive thoughts. Remember, every time you acknowledge yourself, you love yourself a little more.

Nurture Yourself

In the past, often I would take care of myself last and make sure everyone in my family, including the cat and dog, had everything they wanted. When I did get around to thinking of myself, it was usually too late and I was too tired. But recently I have started to do things for myself and feel wonderful about it. It is important to do things for yourself, but it is also important to know what will make you feel wonderful, and what might end up being self-sabotage.

EXERCISE: *How I Nurture Myself*

Take a moment to list some things you can do for yourself that will make you feel good. Notice if it's a real nurture or a cheap thrill: such as having a hot fudge sundae when you have been good on your diet all day, and then beating up on yourself after you do it.

Example:
1. Taking a long bath with bath oil. Putting candles in the bathroom, incense, and soft music while in the tub.
2. Taking a long walk to watch the sunset.
3. Buying flowers for myself.
4. Taking time in the afternoon to have coffee with a friend.
5. Giving myself a hot fudge sun...whoops, that's a potential cheap thrill.
6. Ordering the richest dessert on the menu and eating a few bites.
7. Having a manicure, and if I really feel the need, a pedicure, too.
8. Painting.
9. Going horseback riding.
10. Listening to great music.

YOUR TURN

List things you can do for yourself that will make you feel good.

1. _____

2. _____

3. _____

4. _____

5. _____

6. _____

7. _____

8. _____

9. _____

10. _____

Now start doing some of these things on a daily basis and see how you feel.

Becoming What You Want to Be

Every day in every way you are choosing. You choose what to wear, you choose where you will work. You can choose to believe that you have no choice, that other people are controlling your life, or you can choose to be responsible for your own life and the way you experience it.

All through life you've been making decisions that affect your body and the way it reflects the way you feel inside. You may ignore a backache, deciding it isn't important. The backache may continually worsen until you barely can stand it and you feel awful all the time. Or you may decide to eat only healthy foods so your body will feel wonderful all the time.

Recently, when I became very ill with the flu, I discovered why I have been unable to get my weight under 125 pounds for the past few years. During my illness I lost five pounds, taking my weight down to 120. But when I got on the scale, suddenly I became afraid. During the next week I ate everything in sight, until I gained back the weight. As soon as I weighed 125 pounds again, I felt safe. Then I realized that in my subconscious belief, weighing under 125 pounds brings back all the misery of my former life of suffering, abuse, and addictions. Now that I know that, I can begin to change it.

Each time we learn something new, even if we don't like it, we are one step closer to having the life we want. I used to believe that I would always have fat thighs because fat thighs run in my family. When I realized that fat thighs were merely a belief and I could change that belief, two things happened. First, I was excited that I could change my thighs. Next, I realized that I would have to do something about it. I needed to start by changing my subconscious programming. Instead of thinking, "Everyone in my family has fat thighs, so I must have them also," I began affirming, while I was exercising, "I can have thin, beautiful thighs just because I want them." This was the beginning of the process to change the shape of my thighs. The treasure maps I made contained fabulous-looking, trim thighs. When I looked in the mirror at my legs I said, "I love my thighs; they are lean, toned, and beautiful." Soon my thighs began to look different to me, my clothes fit better and I felt more attractive. I acknowledged my success and continued to follow through, then I added one final step to my MetaFitness program:

Life Chest

In this process, sit quietly with your eyes closed. Visualize a large wooden or metal chest in front of you. Begin to place in the chest all the things you want to have in your life. Visualize yourself with the perfect body, healthy and strong. Visualize your perfect life, with exactly the job and home environment you desire. Visualize your family and friends, your house and car. Those are the kinds of things I put in my life chest; plus, I want financial security. Be very specific if you want to be, or think in general terms. For instance, financial security to me equals a steady, guaranteed income earned by doing what I want to do. I put that thought in the chest. I do not even have to know what work it is I want to do, just that I want to be financially secure. (Next we shoot for wealthy.)

Once you have filled your life chest, close the lid, and while you still have your eyes closed, in your mind, see the chest travel out into the universe. Allow yourself to believe that whatever you sent out in the chest will begin to come true in your life.

Just as you are able to create a picture in your mind of the body you want and the life you want, you can create those things in reality. You are in charge of how your life unfolds. Become aware of how much you bring into your life once you've visualized your desires. Make up the kind of life you want, and then set out to have it come true. Make up the kind of body you want, and use MetaFitness to create it.

Affirmation

I love myself totally.
I have the ability to create the exact body
and life that I want.

APPENDIX
A

SPORTS, ACTIVITIES, AND EXERCISES

"Physical strength can never
permanently withstand the
impact of spiritual force."
— *Franklin D. Roosevelt*

Now that you have nearly finished this book, you may wonder how to continue.

There is a sport or exercise program that works for everybody, but the bottom-line benefit of any form of exercise comes when you do it over the long haul. If you only do it sporadically, it will not work. If you only think about it—unless you are a Zen master—it will not work either. An exercise program is only as good as your willingness to do it.

I suggest you select an exercise program—combining some form of physical activity with affirmations and visualizations—commit to it, and then keep up with it three to six times a week. You may also want to mix and match exercise programs so that you do not run the risk of exercising only one set of muscles, and so you do not get bored.

What about those of you who do not like to exercise at all? The first step here is to begin to want to. Although this may seem like an impossible task, it is not. Begin your program with affirmations and visualizations that encourage you to exercise. For example: "My body is beginning to like to exercise. It feels better and better every day and looks forward to the time I take to move it."

Picture yourself doing some kind of exercise (choose something you think you might like, dancing or tennis perhaps), see yourself smiling and enjoying yourself. Repeat this process often during the day.

The next step is to start doing something you truly enjoy. It may be taking a walk, going for a swim, ballroom dancing, dancing around the house by yourself, joining an aerobics class, playing backyard tag, anything. It does not matter what you choose—just choose something that you like to do, and then do it. If you need a friend to join you, get one.

There is no ONE right way of doing anything. The key is to make exercising pleasant.

The following list of physical activities gives you guidelines to selections that you might choose, the major body parts used for each activity, as well as an affirmation which corresponds both to the actual body part and to what that part represents in your life. You will need to make up your own visualizations. If the sport you love is not here, look up one that is similar and use that affirmation—or make up your own.

You will notice that the primary physical areas used in most activities are the heart and lungs. Where this is the case, I have also included an affirmation for the secondary area used. Since your heart and lungs are probably the most important areas of your body, it is a good idea to become familiar with an affirmation for them regardless of what exercise or activity you choose.

Heart represents: Your center of love and security. Willingness to give and receive love.
Lungs represent: Your ability to take in life.

Affirmation: I love life. I am safe giving and receiving love. My life is filled with love and harmony and I am willing to experience it with joy.

AEROBIC DANCE, REGULAR AEROBICS, AND LOW-IMPACT AEROBICS
Primary Areas: Heart and lungs.
Secondary Areas: Legs, midriff, and arms.

Primary Areas:
Heart represents: Your center of love and security. Willingness to give and receive love.
Lungs represent: Your ability to take in life.

Affirmation: I love life. I am safe giving and receiving love. My life is filled with love and harmony and I am willing to experience it with joy.

Secondary Areas:
 Legs represent: Carrying you forward in life.
 Midriff represents: How you deal with your emotions, with ease or difficulty, with confidence or fear.
 Arms represent: How you embrace life.

Affirmation: I embrace my life and emotions with ease and I move forward with joy and harmony.

Your own affirmation:_____

_____

_____

ARCHERY
 Primary Areas: Eyes, arms, and brain (focus).
 Secondary Areas: Back and midriff.

Primary Areas:
 Eyes represent: Your capacity to see; in this case, to focus and aim your life.
 Arms represent: How you embrace life.
 Brain represents: Your computer that holds all the information. It is your center of activity.

Affirmation: I am focused in life, enjoy my experiences, and embrace life with joy. I am safe with what I know and lovingly operate my mind with ease.

Secondary Areas:
 Back represents: Feeling supported in life.
 Midriff represents: How you deal with your emotions, with ease or difficulty, with confidence or fear.

Affirmation: I am fully supported as I embrace my life, and move forward with ease, enjoying all of my experiences and my emotions.

Your own affirmation:_____

_____

_____

BALLET
Primary Areas: Abdominals and lower back.
Secondary Areas: Legs, midriff, and arms.

Primary Areas:
Abdominals represent: How you assimilate information and your willingness to follow your own knowing.
Lower back represents: Feelings of support, especially financial.

Affirmation: I am supported in my life; all my needs are met in the present time. I take in and easily digest and assimilate new ideas. It is safe for me to listen and to follow my will.

Secondary Areas:
Legs represent: Carrying you forward in life.
Midriff represents: How you deal with your emotions, with ease or difficulty, with confidence or fear.
Arms represent: How you embrace life.

Affirmation: I move forward in life with ease, experience my emotions lightly, and embrace all life's experiences with enthusiasm and joy.

*Your own affirmation:*_____

_____

_____

BASEBALL *(SOFTBALL)*
Primary Areas: Heart and brain (focus).
Secondary Areas: Legs, back, midriff, and arms.

Primary Areas:
Heart represents: Your center of love and security. Willingness to give and receive love.
Brain represents: Your computer that holds all the information. It is your center of all activity.

Affirmation: I love life and I am safe giving and receiving love. It is fun to be the loving operator of my mind. It is easy to be clear and focused.

Secondary Areas:
> **Legs represent:** Carrying you forward in life.
> **Back represents:** Feeling supported in life.
> **Midriff represents:** How you deal with your emotions, with ease or difficulty, with confidence or fear.
> **Arms represent:** How you embrace life.

> *Affirmation: I am fully supported as I embrace my life and move forward with ease, enjoying all of my experiences and my emotions.*

*Your own affirmation:*_____

_____

_____

BASKETBALL
> **Primary Areas:** Heart and lungs.
> **Secondary Areas:** Legs, back, midriff, abdominals, arms, and the brain (focus/coordination).

Primary Areas:
> **Heart represents:** Your center of love and security. Willingness to give and receive love.
> **Lungs represent:** Your ability to take in life.

> *Affirmation: I love life. I am safe giving and receiving love. My life is filled with love and harmony and I am willing to experience it with joy.*

Secondary Areas:
> **Legs represent:** Carrying you forward in life.
> **Back represents:** Feeling supported (or unsupported) in life.
> **Midriff represents:** How you deal with your emotions, with ease or difficulty, with confidence or fear.
> **Abdominals represent:** How you assimilate information and your willingness to follow your own knowing.
> **Arms represent:** How you embrace life.

> *Affirmation: I assimilate each moment and each new idea and am fully supported as I embrace my life and move forward with ease, enjoying all of my experiences and emotions.*

*Your own affirmation:*_____

_____

_____

BELLY DANCING

Primary Areas: Abdominals and lower back.
Secondary Areas: Buttocks, hips, and legs.

Primary Areas:
Abdominals represent: How you assimilate information and your willingness to follow your own knowing.
Lower back represents: Feelings of support, especially financial.

Affirmation: It is safe to take in and assimilate new ideas. I love to fully express my creativity and to follow my own knowing. All my needs are met in present time. I am supported by life and the universe.

Secondary Areas:
Buttocks represent: Your seat of power. They represent how you deal with and experience power (yours and other's).
Hips and pelvic area represent: Balance, movement, and creativity.
Legs represent: Carrying you forward in life.

Affirmation: I am balanced in my power as I move forward in life with ease, expressing my creativity with ease and confidence.

*Your own affirmation:*_____

_____

_____

BICYCLING

Primary Areas: Heart and lungs.
Secondary Area: Legs.

Primary Areas:
Heart represents: Your center of love and security. Willingness to give and receive love.
Lungs represent: Your ability to take in life.

Affirmation: I love life. I am safe giving and receiving love. My life is filled with love and harmony and I am willing to experience it with joy.

Secondary Area:
 Legs represent: Carrying you forward in life.

 Affirmation: I move forward in life with joy and ease. I have total mobility and know all is well wherever I go.

*Your own affirmation:*_____

_____

_____

BOWLING
 Primary Area: Brain (focus).
 Secondary Areas: Back, arms, abdominals.

Primary Area:
 Brain represents: Your computer that holds all the information. It is your center of activity.

 Affirmation: It is fun to be the loving operator of my mind. It is easy to be clear and focused.

Secondary Areas:
 Back represents: Feeling supported in life.
 Arms represent: How you embrace life.
 Abdominals represent: How you assimilate information and your willingness to follow your own knowing.

 Affirmation: I am fully supported as I embrace life and assimilate each moment and each new idea easily and effortlessly.

*Your own affirmation:*_____

_____

_____

BADMINTON
Primary Areas: Heart and lungs.
Secondary Areas: Back, arms, chest, shoulders, midriff, abdominals, and legs.

Primary Areas:
Heart represents: Your center of love and security. Willingness to give and receive love.
Lungs represent: Your ability to take in life.

Affirmation: I love life. I am safe giving and receiving love. My life is filled with love and harmony and I am willing to experience it with joy.

Secondary Areas:
Back represents: Feeling supported in life.
Arms represent: How you embrace life.
Chest represents: Your ability to take in both love and life.
Shoulders represent: How easily you carry your experiences in life.
Midriff represents: How you deal with your emotions, with ease or difficulty, with confidence or fear.
Abdominals represent: How you assimilate information and your willingness to follow your own knowing.
Legs represent: Carrying you forward in life.

Affirmation: I am supported by life as I embrace it fully and take in all my experiences safely and with joy. I give and receive love easily and assimilate new ideas as I carry life with ease and move forward in joy and harmony.

*Your own affirmation:*_____

_____

_____

_____

CANOEING *(KAYAKING)*
Primary Areas: Upper back, shoulders, arms, and chest.
Secondary Areas: Abdominals and lower back.

Primary Areas:
>   **Upper back represents:** Safety and support; guards the heart.
>   **Shoulders represent:** How easily you carry your experiences in life.
>   **Chest represents:** Your ability to take in both love and life.
>   **Arms represent:** How you embrace life.

>   *Affirmation: I am fully supported in life and carry my experiences lightly and with joy. I embrace life with enthusiasm and am safe giving and receiving love. I love life and enjoy life's process.*

Secondary Areas:
>   **Abdominals represent:** How you assimilate information and your willingness to follow your own knowing.
>   **Lower back represents:** Feelings of support, especially financial.

>   *Affirmation: All my needs are met in present time. I am supported in life. I assimilate new ideas and follow my own knowing with confidence.*

*Your own affirmation:*_____

_____

_____

CLIMBING STAIRS
>   **Primary Areas:** Heart and lungs.
>   **Secondary Areas:** Legs, hips, buttocks, and abdominals.

Primary Areas:
>   **Heart represents:** Your center of love and security. Willingness to give and receive love.
>   **Lungs represent:** Your ability to take in life.

>   *Affirmation: I love life. I am safe giving and receiving love. My life is filled with love and harmony and I am willing to experience it with joy.*

Secondary Areas:
>   **Legs represent:** Carrying you forward in life.
>   **Hips and pelvic area represent:** Balance, movement, and creativity.
>   **Buttocks represent:** Your seat of power. They represent how you deal with and experience power (yours and other's).

Abdominals represent: How you assimilate information and your willingness to follow your own knowing.

Affirmation: I move forward in life in balance and harmony, enjoying my power as I assimilate new ideas easily and follow my own knowing with confidence.

*Your own affirmation:*_____

_____

_____

CROSS COUNTRY SKIING *(See SKIING)*

CROQUET
Primary Areas: Back and the brain (focus).
Secondary Area: Arms.

Primary Areas:
Back represents: Feeling supported in life.
Brain represents: Your computer that holds all the information. It is your center of activity.

Affirmation: All my needs are met in present time. I am supported in life. It is fun to be the loving operator of my mind. It is easy to be clear and focused.

Secondary Area:
Arms represent: How you embrace life.

Affirmation: I embrace all of life's experiences with joy and ease.

*Your own affirmation:*_____

_____

_____

DANCE (JAZZ, MODERN, and TAP)
Primary Areas: Heart and lungs.
Secondary Areas: Legs, back, buttocks, abdominals, shoulders, midriff, and arms.

Primary Areas:
Heart represents: Your center of love and security. Willingness to give and receive love.
Lungs represent: Your ability to take in life.

Affirmation: I love life. I am safe giving and receiving love. My life is filled with love and harmony and I am willing to experience it with joy.

Secondary Areas:
Legs represent: Carrying you forward in life.
Back represents: Feeling supported in life.
Buttocks represent: Your seat of power. They represent how you deal with and experience power (yours and other's).
Abdominals represent: How you assimilate information and your willingness to follow your own knowing.
Shoulders represent: How easily you carry your experiences in life.
Midriff represents: How you deal with your emotions, with ease or difficulty, with confidence or fear.
Arms represent: How you embrace life.

Affirmation: I embrace all aspects of my life as I assimilate new ideas and experience my emotions with ease and confidence. I carry my experiences lightly as I move forward joyously, knowing my life fully supports me.

*Your own affirmation:*_____

_____

_____

DIVING
Primary Areas: Brain (focus and balance) and muscles (strength).
Secondary Area: Overall body conditioning.

Primary Areas:
   Brain represents: Your computer that holds all the information. It is your center of activity.
   Muscles represent: Holding the whole structure of your life together. Structure or lack of structure in life.

   Affirmation: It is fun to be the loving operator of my mind. It is easy to be clear and focused. I see life clearly and am able to focus my desires. I have what I need, my life is balanced, structured, and easy to experience.

Secondary Area:
   The entire body represents: How you live your life and feel about yourself.

   Affirmation: I live my life in joy. I am happy and delighted with every day. My life is fun. I enjoy myself, my experiences, and all the people I meet and know. I am loved and accepted wherever I go. I love myself.

Your own affirmation: _____

_____

_____

DOWNHILL SKIING *(See SKIING)*

EXERCISE MACHINES
(depends on which areas you concentrate on)
   Primary Area: The whole body.
   Secondary Area: Whatever you have missed.

Primary Area:
   The whole body represents: Your way of being in the world.

   Affirmation: I love life. It works for me, and it is fun. I am able to see clearly, stay balanced, and enjoy all of my experiences.

Secondary Area:

Whatever you have missed represents: Whatever you are overlooking in your life.

Affirmation: It is easy for me to see and understand all of my life clearly.

*Your own affirmation:*_____

_____

_____

FIELD HOCKEY *(See SOCCER)*

FISHING

Primary Area: Brain.
Secondary Areas: Legs, back, chest, and arms.

Primary Area:

Brain represents: Your computer that holds all the information. It is your center of activity.

Affirmation: I enjoy patience. It comes easily, is restful to my mind, and gives me space to allow things to happen.

Secondary Areas:

Legs represent: Carrying you forward in life.
Back represents: Feeling supported in life.
Chest represents: Your ability to take in both love and life.
Arms represent: How you embrace life.

Affirmation: I embrace life with joy and gratitude as I move forward with ease, fully supported; I am safe in giving and in receiving love.

*Your own affirmation:*_____

_____

_____

GARDENING
Primary Area: Back.
Secondary Areas: Legs and arms.

Primary Area:
Back represents: Feeling supported in life.

Affirmation: I am supported in life. All my needs are met in present time. Life supports me.

Secondary Areas:
Legs represent: Carrying you forward in life.
Arms represent: How you embrace life.

Affirmation: I embrace my life fully, with gratitude and delight as I move forward with ease.

*Your own affirmation:*_____

_____

_____

_____

GOLF
Primary Area: Brain (focus).
Secondary Areas: Back, midriff, legs, chest, and arms.

Primary Area:
Brain represents: Your computer that holds all the information. It is your center of activity.

Affirmation: It is fun to be the loving operator of my mind. It is easy to be clear, focused, and coordinated in all that I do.

Secondary Areas:
Back represents: Feeling supported in life.
Midriff represents: How you deal with your emotions, with ease or difficulty, with confidence or fear.
Chest represents: Your ability to take in both love and life.
Arms represent: How you embrace life.

Affirmation: I embrace life with joy as I move forward with ease. I am safe giving and receiving love. I am secure in my emotions and fully supported.

*Your own affirmation:*_____

_____

_____

GYMNASTICS

Primary Areas: Heart, lungs, and the brain (focus).
Secondary Area: Overall body.

Primary Areas:

Heart represents: Your center of love and security. Willingness to give and receive love.
Lungs represent: Your ability to take in life.
Brain represents: Your computer that holds all the information. It is your center of activity.

Affirmation: I love life. I am safe giving and receiving love. My life is filled with love and harmony and I am willing to experience it with joy. I am the loving operator of my mind and I love coordinating every part of me. It is fun to be the loving operator of my mind. It is easy to be clear, focused, and coordinated in all that I do.

Secondary Area:

The entire body represents: How you live your life and feel about yourself.

Affirmation: I live my life in joy. I am happy and delighted with every day. My life is fun. I enjoy myself, my experiences, and all the people I meet and know. I am loved and accepted wherever I go. I love myself.

*Your own affirmation:*_____

_____

_____

HIKING

Primary Areas: Heart and lungs.
Secondary Areas: Legs, hips, abdominals, and buttocks.

Primary Areas:
Heart represents: Your center of love and security. Willingness to give and receive love.
Lungs represent: Your ability to take in life.

Affirmation: I love life. I am safe giving and receiving love. My life is filled with love and harmony and I am willing to experience it with joy.

Secondary Areas:
Legs represent: Carrying you forward in life.
Hips and pelvic area represent: Balance, movement, and creativity.
Abdominals represent: How you assimilate information and your willingness to follow your own knowing.
Buttocks represent: Your seat of power. They represent how you deal with and experience power (yours and other's).

Affirmation: I assimilate new ideas easily as I move forward in life with joy. Balanced and in harmony, I express my creativity with confidence as I balance all areas of my life with ease.

*Your own affirmation:*_____

_____

_____

HORSEBACK RIDING

Primary Areas: Legs, abdominals, upper back, and lower back.
Secondary Areas: Arms, chest, and shoulders.

Primary Areas:
Legs represent: Carrying you forward in life.
Abdominals represent: How you assimilate information and your willingness to follow your own knowing.
Upper back represents: Safety and support; guards the heart.
Lower back represents: Feelings of support, especially financial.

Affirmation: It is safe for me to let go and move forward in life. I easily take in and assimilate new ideas and am fully supported by my life. I let go and allow my life to flow easily and effortlessly with joy.

Secondary Areas:

Arms represent: How you embrace life.
Chest represents: Your ability to take in both love and life.
Shoulders represent: How easily you carry your experiences in life.

Affirmation: I carry my experiences lightly as I embrace all of life with joy. I live life fully, safely giving and receiving love.

Your own affirmation: _____

_____

_____

_____

HOUSE CLEANING

Primary Area: Back.
Secondary Areas: Shoulders, arms, legs, and abdominals.

Primary Area:

Back represents: Feeling supported in life.

Affirmation: I am supported by life. All my needs are met in present time. I release the past, enjoy the present, and experience order and quiet in my mind.

Secondary Areas:

Shoulders represent: How easily you carry your experiences in life.
Arms represent: How you embrace life.
Legs represent: Carrying you forward in life.
Abdominals represent: How you assimilate information and your willingness to follow your own knowing.

Affirmation: I embrace life fully, carrying my experiences with ease. I assimilate new ideas easily as I move forward in life smoothly and effortlessly.

*Your own affirmation:*_____

_____

_____

ICE SKATING *(See SKATING)*

ICE HOCKEY

   Primary Areas: Heart, lungs, and brain (focus).
   Secondary Areas: Arms and legs.

Primary Areas:
   Heart represents: Your center of love and security. Willingness to give
   and receive love.
   Lungs represent: Your ability to take in life.
   Brain represents: Your computer that holds all the information. It is
   your center of activity.

   *Affirmation: I love life. I am safe giving and receiving love. My life is
   filled with love and harmony and I am willing to experience it
   with joy.*

Secondary Areas:
   Arms represent: How you embrace life.
   Legs represent: Carrying you forward in life.

   *Affirmation: I embrace my life and emotions with ease and I move for-
   ward with joy and harmony.*

*Your own affirmation:*_____

_____

_____

JAZZ DANCE *(See DANCE)*

JOGGING *(See RUNNING)*

MODERN DANCE *(See DANCE)*

PING-PONG

Primary Area: The brain (focus).
Secondary Areas: Back, shoulders, arms, and abdominals.

Primary Area:

Brain represents: Your computer that holds all the information. It is your center of activity.

Affirmation: It is fun to be the loving operator of my mind. It is easy to be clear, focused, and coordinated in all that I do.

Secondary Areas:

Back represents: Feeling supported in life.
Shoulders represent: How easily you carry your experiences in life.
Arms represent: How you embrace life.
Abdominals represent: How you assimilate information and your willingness to follow your own knowing.

Affirmation: I am fully supported by life and embrace it joyously as I take in and assimilate new ideas effortlessly. My life is fun. I carry life lightly and enjoy it greatly.

*Your own affirmation:*_____

_____

_____

RACQUETBALL *(SQUASH)*

Primary Areas: Heart, lungs, and the brain (focus and coordination).
Secondary Areas: Shoulders, back, arms, chest, waist, midriff, abdominals, legs, hips, and buttocks.

Primary Areas:

Heart represents: Your center of love and security. Willingness to give and receive love.
Lungs represent: Your ability to take in life.
Brain represents: Your computer that holds all the information. It is your center of activity.

Affirmation: I love life. I am safe giving and receiving love. My life is filled with love and harmony and I am willing to experience it with joy. It is fun to be the loving operator of my mind. It is easy to be clear, focused, and coordinated in all that I do.

Secondary Areas:
Shoulders represent: How easily you carry your experiences in life.
Back represents: Feeling supported in life.
Arms represent: How you embrace life.
Chest represents: Your ability to take in both love and life.
Waist represents: Your ability to be flexible, to turn easily and see the different angles and sides of life.
Midriff represents: How you deal with your emotions, with ease or difficulty, with confidence or fear.
Abdominals represent: How you assimilate information and your willingness to follow your own knowing.
Legs represent: Carrying you forward in life.
Hips and pelvic area represent: Balance, movement, and creativity.
Buttocks represent: Your seat of power. They represent how you deal with and experience power (yours and other's).

Affirmation: I embrace my life joyously as I move forward with ease, fully supported, balanced, and in harmony. I experience all my emotions with ease. I carry my life lightly and enjoy my power. I assimilate new ideas effortlessly, and trust my own knowing.

*Your own affirmation:*_____

_____

_____

ROLLER SKATING (See SKATING)

ROWING (SCULLING)
Primary Areas: Heart and lungs.
Secondary Areas: Shoulders, arms, back, chest, legs, abdominals, and midriff.

Primary Areas:
Heart represents: Your center of love and security. Willingness to give and receive love.

Lungs represent: Your ability to take in life.

Affirmation: I love life. I am safe giving and receiving love. My life is filled with love and harmony and I am willing to experience it with joy.

Secondary Areas:

Shoulders represent: How easily you carry your experiences in life.
Arms represent: How you embrace life.
Back represents: Feeling supported in life.
Chest represents: Your ability to take in both love and life.
Legs represent: Carrying you forward in life.
Abdominals represent: How you assimilate information and your willingness to follow your own knowing.
Midriff represents: How you deal with your emotions, with ease or difficulty, with confidence or fear.

Affirmation: I embrace life fully as I move forward knowing all is well. I experience my emotions easily, knowing I am safe and in perfect balance giving and receiving love. I release all burdens and know I am fully supported by life.

Your own affirmation: _____

_____

_____

RUNNING *(JOGGING)*

Primary Areas: Heart and lungs.
Secondary Areas: Legs, back, hips, buttocks, and abdominals.

Primary Areas:

Heart represents: Your center of love and security. Willingness to give and receive love.
Lungs represent: Your ability to take in life.

Affirmation: I love life. I am safe giving and receiving love. My life is filled with love and harmony and I am willing to experience it with joy.

Secondary Areas:

Legs represent: Carrying you forward in life.

Back represents: Feeling supported in life.
Hips and pelvic area represent: Balance, movement, and creativity.
Buttocks represent: Your seat of power. They represent how you deal with and experience power (yours and other's).
Abdominals represent: How you assimilate information and your willingness to follow your own knowing.

Affirmation: Assimilating all that is new effortlessly, I move forward in life with ease, fully supported, and balanced in my power.

*Your own affirmation:*_____

_____

_____

SAILING

Primary Areas: Back, shoulders, chest, and arms.
Secondary Areas: Abdominals, legs, hips, and buttocks.

Primary Areas:
Back represents: Feeling supported in life.
Shoulders represent: How easily you carry your experiences in life.
Midriff represents: How you deal with your emotions, with ease or difficulty, with confidence or fear.
Chest represents: Your ability to take in both love and life.
Arms represent: How you embrace life.

Affirmation: I embrace life joyously as I carry my experiences lightly, knowing I am fully supported and safe loving and being loved.

Secondary Areas:
Abdominals represent: How you assimilate information and your willingness to follow your own knowing.
Legs represent: Carrying you forward in life.
Hips and pelvic area represent: Balance, movement, and creativity.
Buttocks represent: Your seat of power. They represent how you deal with and experience power (yours and other's).

Affirmation: Assimilating new ideas easily and effortlessly, I trust my own knowing and enjoy my power as I move forward in life in perfect balance and harmony.

*Your own affirmation:*_____

_____

_____

SCUBA DIVING *(SNORKELING)*
Primary Areas: Legs, hips, and buttocks.
Secondary Areas: Back, shoulders, midriff, and chest.

Primary Areas:
> **Legs represent:** Carrying you forward in life.
> **Hips and pelvic area represent:** Balance, movement, and creativity.
> **Buttocks represent:** Your seat of power. They represent how you deal with and experience power (yours and other's).

> *Affirmation: I am comfortable in my power as I easily move forward in life in perfect balance.*

Secondary Areas:
> **Back represents:** Feeling supported in life.
> **Shoulders represent:** How easily you carry your experiences in life.
> **Midriff represents:** How you deal with your emotions, with ease or difficulty, with confidence or fear.
> **Chest represents:** Your ability to take in both love and life.

> *Affirmation: I experience my emotions with ease as I take in and give out love and nourishment in perfect balance. Fully supported and safe in my life, I carry my experiences lightly and easily.*

*Your own affirmation:*_____

_____

_____

SCULLING *(See ROWING)*

SKATING *(ICE and ROLLER SKATING)*
> **Primary Areas:** Heart and lungs.
> **Secondary Areas:** Legs, hips, buttocks, back, midriff, and abdominals.

Primary Areas:

Heart represents: Your center of love and security. Willingness to give and receive love.
Lungs represent: Your ability to take in life.

Affirmation: I love life. I am safe giving and receiving love. My life is filled with love and harmony and I am willing to experience it with joy.

Secondary Areas:

Legs represent: Carrying you forward in life.
Hips and pelvic area represent: Balance, movement, and creativity.
Back represents: Feeling supported in life.
Midriff represents: How you deal with your emotions, with ease or difficulty, with confidence or fear.
Abdominals represent: How you assimilate information and your willingness to follow your own knowing.

Affirmation: Accepting my power, I move forward in life easily, balanced, and in perfect harmony. I assimilate new ideas with ease and experience my emotions lightly, knowing I am fully supported by life.

*Your own affirmation:*_____

_____

_____

SKIING *(CROSS-COUNTRY and DOWNHILL)*

Primary Areas: Heart and lungs.
Secondary Areas: Legs, hips, buttocks, midriff, arms, shoulders, back, and abdominals.

Primary Areas:

Heart represents: Your center of love and security. Willingness to give and receive love.
Lungs represent: Your ability to take in life.

Affirmation: I love life. I am safe giving and receiving love. My life is filled with love and harmony and I am willing to experience it with joy.

Secondary Areas:

Legs represent: Carrying you forward in life.

Hips and pelvic area represent: Balance, movement, and creativity.

Buttocks represent: Your seat of power. They represent how you deal with and experience power (yours and other's).

Midriff represents: How you deal with your emotions, with ease or difficulty, with confidence or fear.

Arms represent: How you embrace life.

Shoulders represent: How easily you carry your experiences in life.

Back represents: Feeling supported in life.

Abdominals represent: How you assimilate information and your willingness to follow your own knowing.

Affirmation: I embrace life joyously as I move forward easily, in perfect balance and harmony. I shoulder my experiences with ease, accepting my power and assimilating new ideas effortlessly. I am fully supported by life.

*Your own affirmation:*_____

_____

_____

SNORKELING *(See SCUBA DIVING)*

SOFTBALL *(See BASEBALL)*

SOCCER *(FIELD HOCKEY)*

Primary Areas: Heart, lungs, and brain (focus).

Secondary Areas: Legs, hips, upper back, shoulders, arms, and buttocks.

Primary Areas:

Heart represents: Your center of love and security. Willingness to give and receive love.

Lungs represent: Your ability to take in life.

Brain represents: Your computer that holds all the information. It is your center of activity.

Affirmation: I love life. I am safe giving and receiving love. My life is filled with love and harmony and I am willing to experience it with joy. It is fun to be the loving operator of my mind. It is easy to be clear, focused, and coordinated in all that I do.

Secondary Areas:

Legs represent: Carrying you forward in life.

Hips and pelvic area represent: Balance, movement, and creativity.

Buttocks represent: Your seat of power. They represent how you deal with and experience power (yours and other's).

Upper back represents: Safety and support; guards the heart.

Shoulders represent: How easily you carry your experiences in life.

Arms represent: How you embrace life.

Affirmation: I am comfortable in my power as I easily move forward in life in perfect balance.

*Your own affirmation:*_____

_____

_____

SPEED-WALKING

Primary Areas: Heart and lungs.

Secondary Areas: Legs, hips, buttocks, waist, abdominals, midriff, arms, chest, and back.

Primary Areas:

Heart represents: Your center of love and security. Willingness to give and receive love.

Lungs represent: Your ability to take in life.

Affirmation: I love life. I am safe giving and receiving love. My life is filled with love and harmony and I am willing to experience it with joy.

Secondary Areas:

Legs represent: Carrying you forward in life.

Hips and pelvic area represent: Balance, movement, and creativity.

Buttocks represent: Your seat of power. They represent how you deal with and experience power (yours and other's).

Waist represents: Your ability to be flexible, to turn easily and see the different angles and sides of life.
Abdominals represent: How you assimilate information and your willingness to follow your own knowing.
Midriff represents: How you deal with your emotions, with ease or difficulty, with confidence or fear.
Arms represent: How you embrace life.
Chest represents: Your ability to take in both love and life.
Back represents: Feeling supported in life.

Affirmation: I am balanced and secure as I move forward in life with great flexibility. Assimilating new ideas easily, I accept my power and handle my emotions effortlessly. I am fully supported by life and am safe giving and receiving love and nourishment.

*Your own affirmation:*_____

_____

_____

SQUASH *(See RACQUETBALL)*

SWIMMING
Primary Area: Your whole body.

Primary Area:
The entire body represents: How you live your life and feel about yourself.

Affirmation: I live my life in joy. I am happy and delighted with every day. My life is fun. I enjoy myself, my experiences, and all the people I meet and know. I am loved and accepted wherever I go. I love myself.

*Your own affirmation:*_____

_____

_____

TAP DANCING *(See DANCE)*

TENNIS

Primary Areas: Heart, lungs, and brain (focus).
Secondary Areas: Arms, shoulders, chest, back, midriff, waist, hips, buttocks, and legs.

Primary Areas:
Heart represents: Your center of love and security. Willingness to give and receive love.
Lungs represent: Your ability to take in life.
Brain represents: Your computer that holds all the information. It is your center of activity.

Affirmation: I love life. I am safe giving and receiving love. My life is filled with love and harmony and I am willing to experience it with joy. It is fun to be the loving operator of my mind. It is easy to be clear, focused, and coordinated in all that I do.

Secondary Areas:
Arms represent: How you embrace life.
Shoulders represent: How easily you carry your experiences in life.
Chest represents: Your ability to take in both love and life.
Back represents: Feeling supported in life.
Midriff represents: How you deal with your emotions, with ease or difficulty, with confidence or fear.
Waist represents: Your ability to be flexible, to turn easily and see the different angles and sides of life.
Hips and pelvic area represent: Balance, movement, and creativity.
Buttocks represent: Your seat of power. They represent how you deal with and experience power (yours and other's).
Legs represent: Carrying you forward in life.

Affirmation: Balanced and in harmony I move forward in life with joy, embracing all of my experiences and emotions easily and effortlessly. Fully supported I carry life lightly, safely giving and receiving love. I happily own my power. Seeing all sides of a situation, I am able to turn in any direction with ease.

*Your own affirmation:*_____

_____

_____

VOLLEYBALL

Primary Areas: Heart, lungs, and brain (focus).
Secondary Areas: Arms, shoulders, back, and chest.

Primary Areas:

Heart represents: Your center of love and security. Willingness to give and receive love.
Lungs represent: Your ability to take in life.
Brain represents: Your computer that holds all the information. It is your center of activity.

Affirmation: I love life. I am safe giving and receiving love. My life is filled with love and harmony and I am willing to experience it with joy.

Secondary Areas:

Arms represent: How you embrace life.
Shoulders represent: How easily you carry your experiences in life.
Back represents: Feeling supported in life.
Chest represents: Your ability to take in both love and life.

Affirmation: I carry my experiences lightly as I fully embrace life with ease. I am supported by life and I am safe giving and receiving love and nourishment.

*Your own affirmation:*_____

_____

_____

WALKING

Primary Areas: Heart and lungs.
Secondary Areas: Legs, hips, buttocks, and abdominals.

Primary Areas:

Heart represents: Your center of love and security. Willingness to give and receive love.
Lungs represent: Your ability to take in life.

Affirmation: I love life. I am safe giving and receiving love. My life is filled with love and harmony and I am willing to experience it with joy.

Secondary Areas:
   Legs represent: Carrying you forward in life.
   Hips and pelvic area represent: Balance, movement, and creativity.
   Buttocks represent: Your seat of power. They represent how you deal with and experience power (yours and other's).
   Abdominals represent: How you assimilate information and your willingness to follow your own knowing.

   Affirmation: Balanced and in harmony, I easily and effortlessly move forward in life. I assimilate new ideas with ease, enjoying my power and the power of others.

*Your own affirmation:*_____

_____

_____

WATER-SKIING
   Primary Areas: Abdominals, back, and legs.
   Secondary Areas: Shoulders, chest, and arms.

Primary Areas:
   Abdominals represent: How you assimilate information and your willingness to follow your own knowing.
   Back represents: Feeling supported in life.
   Legs represent: Carrying you forward in life.

   Affirmation: I carry my experiences lightly as I fully embrace life with ease. I am supported by life and I am safe giving and receiving love and nourishment.

Secondary Areas:
   Shoulders represent: How easily you carry your experiences in life.
   Chest represents: Your ability to take in both love and life.
   Arms represent: How you embrace life.

   Affirmation: Balanced and in harmony I move forward in life with joy, embracing all of my experiences and emotions easily and effortlessly. Fully supported, I carry life lightly, safely giving and receiving love.

*Your own affirmation:*_____

_____

_____

A P P E N D I X
B

ONCE OVER LIGHTLY

"If we rebuild our physical selves, there is a lot we can do. . . . Strong and painless, we will be able to change our world for the better.
— *Bonnie Prudden*

Although MetaFitness is not a formal exercise program, it does not automatically exclude traditional exercise movements. This chapter is designed for those of you who like to follow a structured exercise routine. The following exercises will help you understand how to use affirmations along with your body movements. Repetition of the affirmations while you exercise will enhance the progress you make, more quickly changing your body and your life.

HEAD ROLLS

For the neck, which represents balance and flexibility.

Stand with your feet apart, hands resting at your sides. Tighten your buttocks and abdominals, continue to breathe normally. Slowly lower your head forward and begin to circle, first over your right shoulder, back, over your left shoulder, and forward again. Now circle head in the other direction, over your left shoulder, back, over your right shoulder, and forward again. Do this exercise eight times and repeat the affirmation: *"I am flexible. I see all viewpoints of life. I love my neck."*

SHOULDER CIRCLES

For the shoulders, which represent that which carries and supports, and how we carry our experiences in life, as burdens or with joy.

Stand with your feet apart, hands resting at your sides. Tighten your buttocks and abdominals and breathe normally. Slowly circle both shoulders forward, up, back, and down. Repeat four times. Now circle back, up, forward, and down. Repeat four times. Do this series twice and repeat the affirmation:

"I release all burdens. I shoulder my experiences with ease. I love my shoulders."

ARM TWISTS

For the arms, which represent how we embrace and hold the experiences of life.

Stand with your feet apart, your hands resting at your sides. Tighten your buttocks and abdominals and breathe normally. Raise your right arm out to the side to shoulder height and bend it slightly. Keeping your elbow slightly bent twist arm under until palm faces upward. Now twist arm up so that palm faces upward. Repeat twisting eight times and change arms. Do series twice and repeat the affirmation:

"I have the ability and the capacity to embrace and hold my life with joy. I love my arms."

WRIST CIRCLES

For the wrists, which represent movement and ease.

Stand with your feet apart, hands resting at your sides. Tighten your buttocks and abdominals and breathe normally. Bend both elbows and raise both forearms in front of you. Turn palms up. Slowly circle both wrists up, inward, down, and outward eight times. Now turn palms down and circle wrists down, in, up, and outward again. Repeat eight times and do series twice while you repeat the affirmation:

"I handle all my experiences with wisdom, love, joy, and ease. I love my wrists."

OPEN AND CLOSE

For the hands, which represent how we hold or clutch our experiences in life.

Stand with your feet apart, hands resting at your sides. Tighten your buttocks and abdominals and breathe normally. Bend both elbows and raise both forearms in front of you. Turn palms up. Slowly clench hands into a fist. Now open hands, stretching fingers as far as possible. Do this eight times while you repeat the affirmation:

"I hold each experience easily and effortlessly. I love my hands."

PRONE ARM LIFTS

For the upper back, which guards the heart and represents support.

Lie on the floor on your stomach. Stretch your body full out with your forehead resting on the floor and your arms stretched over your head. Breathe normally. Keeping your head down and your arms straight and close to your ears, raise first your right arm up and then your left. Do this eight times while you repeat the affirmation:

"I am safe and supported. I carry joy and move with ease. I love my back."

WASHING MACHINE

For the middle back, which represents feelings of guilt and being stuck in the "gunk" of life.

Stand with your feet apart. Tighten your buttocks and abdominals and breathe normally. Raise your bent elbows to forty-five degree angles from your sides and bend forward from your hips. Now twist your upper body back and forth like the motions of a washing machine. Pull your elbow back each time you twist upward. Do this sixteen times and say the affirmation:

"I release the past. I am free to move forward with joy and ease. I love my back."

ARCH AND FLATTEN

For the lower back, which represents feelings of support, in this case having to do with finances and "real" property.

Lie on your back on the floor. Bend your arms and place your hands parallel to your head. Bend your knees and place your feet on the floor. Keeping your upper back and your buttocks on the floor, slowly arch your lower back. Hold it in the arched position for two seconds and flatten it against the floor. Hold this flattened position, with your entire spine on the floor, for four seconds. Do the arch and flatten eight times and repeat the affirmation:

"I trust and am supported by life. I always have what I need. I love my back."

SNAP AND STRETCH

For the chest, which houses the heart and lungs and represents your ability to take in both love and life. It represents your ability to feel safe giving and receiving love.

Stand with your feet apart. Tighten your buttocks and abdominals and raise both arms to shoulder height. Bend your elbows and, keeping them pointed outward, bring both hands together to meet in front of your chest.

Keeping elbows bent, pull (snap) both arms backward to open your chest. Now bring hands together again. This time, straighten your arms, turn your palms upward, and pull both straight arms backward to stretch and open your chest. Bend your elbows and bring both hands together in front of your chest again. Do this sixteen times and repeat the affirmation:

"I take in and give out nourishment and love in perfect balance. I love my chest."

PUSH-PULL

For the breasts, which represent nurturing of self and others.

Stand with your feet apart. Tighten your buttocks and abdominals. Raise both bent arms up to shoulder height and, keeping elbows pointed outward, clasp your hands in front of your chest in an overhand/underhand grip. Holding your hands together, pull your arms outward, creating resistance in your arms. Now place the heels of your hands together and push arms inward, again creating resistance. Do this eight times and repeat the affirmation:

"I am balanced in giving and receiving love. I nurture myself and others equally. I love my breasts."

ARM SWINGS

For the midriff, which represents how you deal with your emotions, with ease or difficulty, with confidence or fear.

Stand with your feet apart. Tighten your buttocks and abdominals and breathe normally. Raise both arms to the right and, keeping your hips still, twist your torso to the right. Now swing your arms to the left and twist your torso to the left. Keep your feet flat on the floor, your hips still, and follow the motion of your arms with your head. Do this sixteen times and say the affirmation:

"I am safe feeling all of my emotions. I am strong and capable and I love my midriff."

TORSO TWISTS

For the waist, which represents your ability to turn easily and be flexible in the way you move in your life.

Stand with your feet apart, your hands resting at your sides. Tighten your buttocks and abdominals and breathe normally. Bend your arms and raise them to shoulder height. Twist your torso back and forth, like a washing machine agitating, sixteen times and repeat the affirmation:

"I am able to turn any direction in life with joy and ease. My waist is toned, smooth, and flexible."

CRUNCHES

For the stomach, which represents how you hold nourishment and digest new ideas. It houses your creativity and your will.

Lie on the floor on your back. Bend your knees, put your feet flat on the floor, and place your hands behind your neck. In small "crunching" motions, raise and lower your back off the floor, pulling your chest toward your bent legs. Each time you raise your back off the floor, breathe out; each time you lower your back, breathe in. Repeat sixteen times and say the affirmation:

"I digest life with ease. I am safe to fully experience all that I create and all that comes to me in my life. I love my stomach."

HIP LIFT

For the hips, which represent balance, movement, and creativity.

Stand with your feet slightly apart and hands resting at your sides. Tighten your buttocks and abdominals and breathe normally. Turn your right foot inward and lift your right hip upward. Twist your hip forward as if you wanted to see dust on your right buttock. Lower your hip and turn your foot outward. Repeat eight times and change legs. Repeat eight times with left leg. Do series twice and say the affirmation:

"I am free to move forward, in perfect balance, with joy and laughter. I love my hips."

PRONE LEG LIFTS

For the buttocks, which represent the seat of power and represent how you deal with power, yours and other people's.

Lie on your stomach on the floor with your legs stretched out and your head resting on your arms which are bent under you. Turn your face to the side, be comfortable, and breathe normally. Tighten your buttocks and abdominals. Keep your legs straight and your hip bones on the floor and raise your right leg up. Hold it up for two seconds and lower it. Raise your left leg up. Hold it up for two seconds and lower it. Do this series eight times and say the affirmation:

"I accept my power. I use my power with wisdom. I love my buttocks."

LEG SWINGS

For the thighs, which represent strength and forward motion. They also hold childhood guilt and anger, especially pertaining to father-daughter relationships.

Lie on your right side. Rest on your right elbow and forearm and place your left hand on the floor in front of you. Tighten your buttocks and abdominals and breathe normally.

Swing your right leg forward and back twice and then circle it slowly forward, up, back, and down twice. Repeat once and turn over to your left side. Repeat entire exercise with left leg.

Turn over to your right side again, and this time swing your leg back and forward twice, then circle it slowly back, up, forward, and down twice. Repeat on your left side and do the entire series twice while you say the affirmation:

"I forgive all childhood trespasses, real and imagined, and move forward in my life with strength and ease. I love my thighs."

PLIÉS

For the knees, which represent pride and ego, and balance and flexibility. Stand with your feet apart and turned slightly outward, your hands raised slightly in front of you. Tighten your buttocks and abdominals and breathe normally. Slowly bend your knees halfway down and hold for two seconds. Slowly return to standing. Create resistance in your legs so that you feel your legs working. Repeat twelve times while you say the affirmation:

"My life is balanced. I work and I play equally, with equal joy and delight. I bend and flow with ease. I love my knees."

ROCKING BACK AND FORTH

For the calves, which represent carrying us forward in life.

Stand with your feet together, hands resting by your sides. Tighten your buttocks and abdominals and breathe normally. Keeping your abdominals tight, rock forward and raise yourself slowly up onto the balls of your feet. Hold two seconds, return your heels to the floor and slowly rock backward to lift your toes and the balls of your feet off the floor. Hold two seconds. Continue to rock forward and back slowly (be sure to go all the way up onto the balls of your feet) twelve times and say the affirmation:

"I move forward in my life safely and with ease. I am safe now and in the future. I love my calves."

KNEE WAG

For the ankles, which represent the ability to take in and receive pleasure, inflexibility and guilt.

Stand with your feet slightly apart, your hands raised slightly in front of you. Tighten your buttocks and abdominals and breathe normally. Bend your knees slightly and push them to the right. Allow your ankles to bend so that you lean on the outside of your right foot, the inside of your left. Now shift your knees to the left, bending your ankles and leaning on the outside of your left foot, the inside of your right. Shift back and forth sixteen times and say the affirmation:

"I am safe. I move with ease and flexibility and communicate freely. All is well with me in the world. I love my ankles."

CURL AND FLATTEN

For the feet, which represent our base, our roots, and the quality of our way of being in the world.

Stand with your feet together and hands resting at your sides. Tighten your buttocks and abdominals and breathe normally. Curl your feet inward so that you are leaning on the outside of both feet and there is a space between your arches. Hold two seconds and flatten. Now lift your toes upward and hold two seconds. Return to flat foot position. Do the curl and flatten twelve times and say the affirmation:

"I love my life the way I choose to live. I am safe following my dreams; I love taking care of myself; all is well and perfect in my life. I love my feet."

PICK UP PENCILS

For the toes, which represent the minor details of the future.

Sit in a chair. Place a pencil or a small rubber ball by your bare feet. Start with your right foot. Pick up the object with your toes (place the pencil or the ball between the toes and the ball of your foot, scrunch your toes under, and lift up). Release the object and do this four times. Change feet and do this four times. Repeat the affirmation:

"All details take care of themselves; it is safe for me to let go. I love my toes."

FORWARD STRETCHES

For flexibility, which represents just that—how flexible you are in life.

Sit on the floor with your feet together and legs outstretched in front of you. Keeping your back and legs straight, bend forward and stretch your hands toward your feet. Hold this position and pulse gently eight times. Now, continuing to hold your legs straight, round your back and pulse your head gently toward your knees eight times. Sit straight again, shake out your legs, and repeat the series one more time as you say the affirmation:

"I am flexible. I move in my life and in my body with grace and fluidity. I love the way I move."

CELLULITE MASSAGE

Represents stored anger, rage, unhappiness, and disappointment. It also represents self-denial and self-punishment.

It is best to do cellulite massage without clothes on. Sit on the floor or in a chair. Take hold of the outside of your right thigh with both hands in a pinching hold. Move your hands back and forth, holding onto the pinch of flesh, in an S-curve motion. Repeat a few times and move to another area to hold. Work the whole outside of your thigh from the hip to the knee and the inside of your thigh from the knee to about six inches above your knee. Also the front and back of your thigh, your buttocks and hips, and anywhere else you notice cellulite. Do not massage the inside of your thigh in this manner. Repeat this massage (as if you were kneading bread) for three to five minutes on each leg, buttock, and hip and say:

"I love my body. I release all anger, rage, disappointment, and unhappiness, real and imagined, and go forth in joy and happiness. I joyously allow myself to have the life I want."

Sample Movements with Affirmations

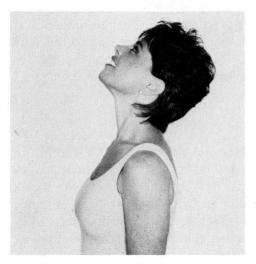

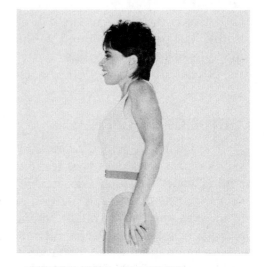

HEAD ROLLS

Affirmation:
I am flexible. I see all viewpoints of life. I love my neck.

SHOULDER CIRCLES:

Affirmation:
I release all burdens. I shoulder my experiences with ease. I love my shoulders.

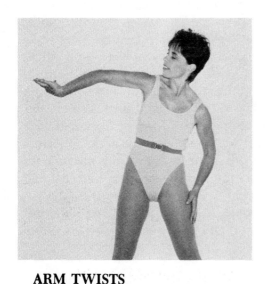

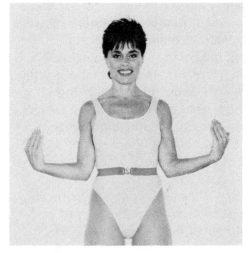

ARM TWISTS

Affirmation:
I have the ability and capacity to embrace and hold my life with joy. I love my arms.

WRIST CIRCLES

Affirmation:
I handle all my experiences with wisdom, love, joy and ease. I love my wrists.

Sample Movements with Affirmations

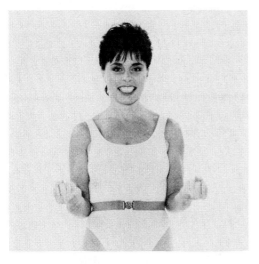

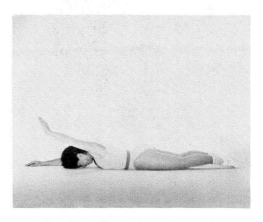

OPEN AND CLOSE

Affirmation:
I hold each experience easily and effortlessly. I love my hands.

PRONE ARM LIFTS

Affirmation:
I am safe and supported. I carry joy and move with ease. I love my upper back.

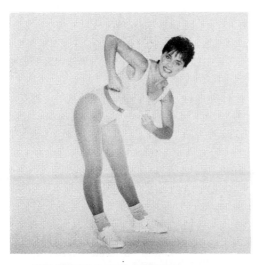

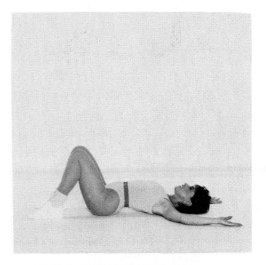

WASHING MACHINE

Affirmation:
I release the past. I am free to move forward with joy and ease. I love my middle back.

ARCH AND FLATTTEN

Affirmation:
I trust life and am supported by life. I always have what I need. I love my lower back.

Sample Movements with Affirmations

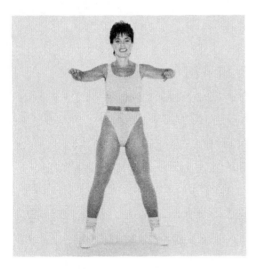

SNAP AND STRETCH

Affirmation:
I take in and give out nourishment and love in perfect balance. I love my chest.

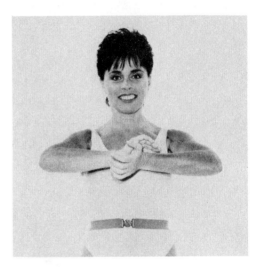

PUSH-PULL

Affirmation:
I am balanced in giving and receiving love. I nurture myself and others equally. I love my breasts.

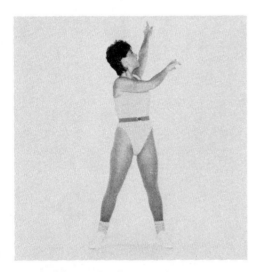

ARM SWINGS

Affirmation:
I am safe feeling all of my emotions. I am strong and capable and I love my midriff.

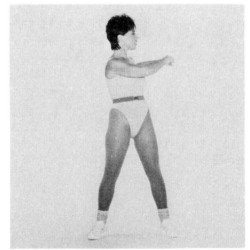

TORSO TWISTS

Affirmation:
I am able to turn any direction in life with joy and ease. My waist is toned, smooth, and flexible. I love my waist.

Sample Movements with Affirmations

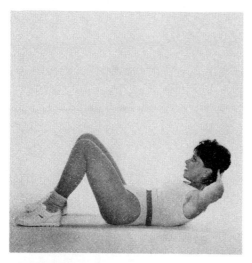

CRUNCHES

Affirmation:
I digest life with ease. I am safe to fully experience all that I create and all that comes to me in my life. I love my stomach.

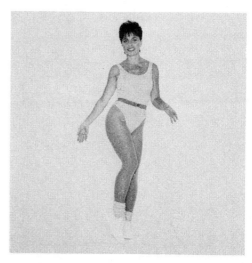

HIP LIFT

Affirmation:
I am free as I move forward, in perfect balance, with joy and laughter. I love my hips.

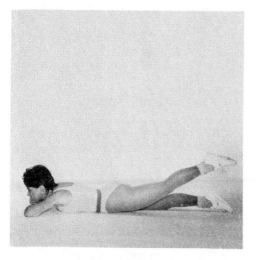

PRONE LEG LIFTS

Affirmation:
I accept my power. I use my power with wisdom. I love my buttocks.

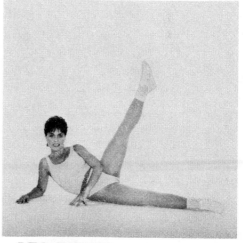

LEG SWINGS

Affirmation:
I forgive all my childhood trespasses, real or imagined. I move forward in my life with strength and ease. I love my thighs.

Sample Movements with Affirmations

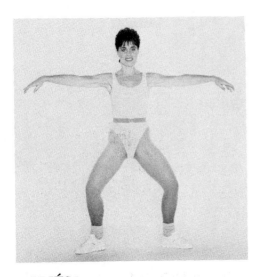

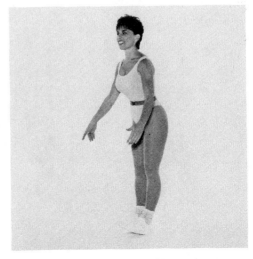

PLIÉS

Affirmation:
My life is balanced. I work and
play equally, with joy and delight.
I bend and flow with ease.
I love my knees.

ROCKING BACK AND FORTH

Affirmation:
I move forward in my life safely and
with ease. I am safe now and in the
future. I love my calves.

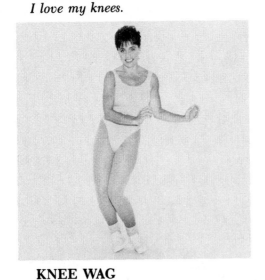

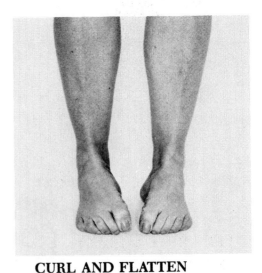

KNEE WAG

Affirmation:
I am safe. I move with ease and
flexibility and communicate freely.
All is well with me in the world.
I love my ankles.

CURL AND FLATTEN

Affirmation:
I love my life the way I choose to
live. I am safe following my dreams.
I love taking care of myself. I love
my feet.

Sample Movements with Affirmations

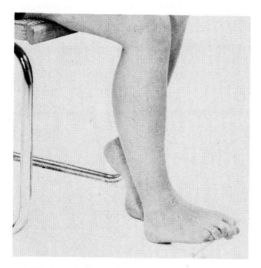

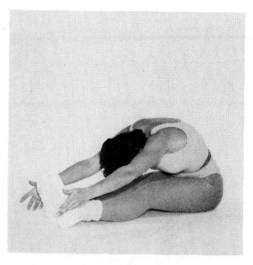

PICK UP PENCILS
Affirmation:
All details take care of themselves.
It is safe for me to let go. I love
my toes.

FORWARD STRETCHES
Affirmation:
I am flexible. I move in my life and
in my body with grace and fluidity.
I love the way I move.

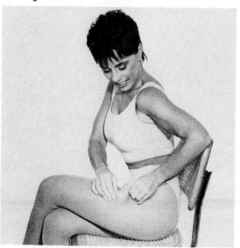

CELLULITE MASSAGE
Affirmation:
I love my body. I release all anger,
rage, disappointment, and unhappi-
ness, real or imagined, and go forth
in joy and happiness. I joyously
allow myself to have the life I want.

APPENDIX
C

Suggested Reading and Workshops

SUGGESTED READING

Bach, Richard *Bridge Across Forever*
Bach, Richard *Illusions: The Adventures of a Reluctant Messiah*
Bach, Richard *Jonathan Livingston Seagull*
Bach, Richard *One*
Boone, J. Allen *Kinship with All Life*
Bolen, Jean *Goddesses in Everywoman: A New Psychology of Women*
Campbell, Joseph, and Bill Moyers *The Power of Myth*
Carey, Ken *Vision*
Castenada, Carlos *Journey to Ixtlan*
Castenada, Carlos *Separate Reality*
Castenada, Carlos *Tales of Power*
Castenada, Carlos *Teachings of Don Juan*
Gawain, Shakti *Creative Visualization*
Gawain, Shakti *Living in the Light*
Gershon, David, and Gail Straub
    Empowerment: The Art of Creating Your Life As You Want It
Hay, Louise L. *Heal Your Body*
Hay, Louise L. *I Love My Body*
Hay, Louise L. *You Can Heal Your Life*
Hill, Napoleon *Think and Grow Rich*

Jampolsky, Gerald G. *Goodbye to Guilt: Releasing Fear Through Forgiveness*

Jampolsky, Gerald G. *Love Is Letting Go of Fear*

Jampolsky, Gerald G. *Teach Only Love: The Seven Principles of Attitudinal Healing*

Keyes, Ken, Jr. *A Conscious Person's Guide to Relationships*

Keyes, Ken, Jr. *Handbook to Higher Consciousness*

Laut, Phil *Money Is My Friend*

Millman, Dan *Way of the Peaceful Warrior: A Book That Changes Lives*

Norwood, Robin *Women Who Love Too Much*

Peck, M. Scott *The Road Less Traveled*

Ponder, Catherine *The Dynamic Laws of Prosperity*

Ponder, Catherine *The Healing Secrets of the Ages*

Schwartz, Bob *Diets Don't Work*

Ray, Sondra *I Deserve Love*

Ray, Sondra *Loving Relationships*

Ray, Sondra *The Only Diet There Is*

Shinn, Florence S. *The Game of Life and How to Play It*

Shinn, Florence S. *The Power of the Spoken Word*

Shinn, Florence S. *The Secret Door to Success*

Verny, Thomas, and John Kelly *The Secret Life of the Unborn Child*

SUGGESTED WORKSHOPS

Empowerment Workshop David Gershon and Gail Straub (West Hurley, New York)

The Forum (formerly est) given at "Area Centers" nationally; headquarters (San Francisco, California)

Let Go and Live June Graham and Jim Spencer (New York, New York)

Love Yourself, Heal Your Life Workshop Louise L. Hay, Louise L. Hay Educational Institute (Santa Monica, California)

Loving Relationships Training (LRT) Sondra Ray, given nationally; headquarters (New York, New York)

NLP (Neuro-Linguistic Programming) given nationally

Self-Esteem Workshop Cherie Carter-Scott, given nationally, Motivation Management Services (Los Angeles, California)

Silva Mind Control given nationally

Technologies for Creating (formerly DMA) headquarters (Salem, Massachusetts)

Warrior-Healer Workshop Tim Piering and Coneley Falk (Los Angeles, California)

SUGGESTED WORKSHOP SPONSORS

Esalen Institute (Big Sur, California)

Interface (Boston, Massachusetts)

Omega Institute (Rhinebeck, New York)

For More Information
Detach and Return Reply Card

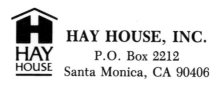

HAY HOUSE, INC.
P.O. Box 2212
Santa Monica, CA 90406

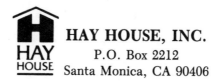

HAY HOUSE, INC.
P.O. Box 2212
Santa Monica, CA 90406

Look for Suzy's Meta Fitness, body/mind workout video, audio and subliminal audio in your local bookstores. Or write or call (213) 394-7445 for our FREE catalog with a complete listing of Hay House products.

Name_____

Address_____

_____

Look for Suzy's Meta Fitness, body/mind workout video, audio and subliminal audio in your local bookstores. Or write or call (213) 394-7445 for our FREE catalog with a complete listing of Hay House products.

Name_____

Address_____

_____